Reducing Adverse Drug Events

BREAKTHROUGH SERIES Guide

Reducing
Adverse Drug Events

Lucian L. Leape

Andrea Kabcenell

Donald M. Berwick

Jane Roessner

INSTITUTE FOR
HEALTHCARE
IMPROVEMENT

Although the editorial process for the Institute for Healthcare Improvement's Breakthrough Series Guides is extensive, readers are cautioned not to base their clinical, diagnostic, therapeutic, or drug dosage choices or actions solely on information presented in the Guide.

Institute for Healthcare Improvement
135 Francis Street
Boston, MA 02215
(617) 754-4800

Breakthrough Series Guides
Managing Editor: Penny Carver, MEd
Design and Composition: Codesign, Boston

Reducing Adverse Drug Events
Authors:
Lucian L. Leape, MD
Andrea Kabcenell, RN, MPH
Donald M. Berwick, MD
Jane Roessner, PhD

First Edition
Printed in the USA
10 9 8 7 6 5 4 3

Library of Congress Catalog
Card Number: 98-070033

ISBN 1-890070-03-3

INSTITUTE FOR
HEALTHCARE
IMPROVEMENT

The Institute for Healthcare Improvement (IHI) is a nonprofit organization founded in 1991. The Institute is designed to be a major force for integrative and collaborative efforts to accelerate improvement in the health care systems of the United States and Canada. The Institute provides bridges connecting people and organizations committed to real reforms, who believe they can accomplish more together than they can separately.

In addition to the Breakthrough Series, IHI conducts courses, the annual National Forum on Quality Improvement in Health Care, networks of health care organizations engaged in change, and research and demonstration projects in regulation and professional education reform.

For more information about Breakthrough Series activities and publications, as well as other programs and activities sponsored by the Institute for Healthcare Improvement, please call (617) 754-4800, fax (617) 754-4848, or write to IHI, 135 Francis Street, Boston, MA 02215.

Donald M. Berwick, MD
President and CEO
Institute for Healthcare Improvement

ABOUT THE BREAKTHROUGH SERIES

The Institute for Healthcare Improvement developed the Breakthrough Series to bring together groups of health care organizations that share a commitment to making major, rapid changes that will produce breakthrough results: lower cost and better outcomes at the same time.

Each Collaborative in the Breakthrough Series includes 20 to 40 health care organizations. Focusing on a single topic, these organizations study the latest scientific information on improving a specific clinical or operational area and learn effective means to put that information into practice for rapid improvement.

Breakthrough Series topics are chosen because they are ripe for improvement:

- Substantial knowledge exists about how to achieve better performance.
- There is a gap between the best available knowledge and everyday practice.
- Strong examples exist of some organizations (even if only a few) that have already applied that knowledge and "broken through" to unprecedented results.
- Improvement responds to the social need to reduce the cost of health care, achieve better clinical outcomes, and increase patient satisfaction.

BREAKTHROUGH SERIES GUIDES

Published Volumes

Reducing Delays and Waiting Times Throughout the Healthcare System

Improving Asthma Care in Children and Adults

Reducing Adverse Drug Events

Reducing Cesarean Section Rates While Maintaining Maternal and Infant Outcomes

Reducing Costs and Improving Outcomes in Adult Intensive Care

Forthcoming Volumes

Improving Outcomes and Reducing Costs in Adult Cardiac Surgery

Providing More Effective Care for Low Back Pain

Improving Prescribing Practices

Improving Care for People with Chronic Conditions

Improving Service in Health Care

The Breakthrough Series Guides are designed for health care leaders and practitioners who want to make change.

When do you need a guide? When you want to go somewhere you've never been before or learn how to do something you've never done before. Guides can also be useful when you're returning to a place you've already visited. Whether you are just beginning to work on reducing adverse drug events or returning to the effort, you will benefit from this Guide.

What do you need in a guide? Clear explanations, useful tips, and step-by-step instruction—so that you can learn as quickly as possible. Practical and user-friendly, the Breakthrough Series Guides are based on the real experiences of health care organizations that have made significant improvements. The aim of the Guides is to disseminate as widely as possible what these organizations have learned, in order to help others design and implement their own breakthrough improvements.

Contents

Acknowledgments

Thanks to the organizations that took part in the Breakthrough Series Collaborative on Reducing Adverse Drug Events. They made a commitment to making major, rapid improvements in their organizations. They shared generously their insights, successes, and lessons learned; in so doing, they have paved a path that many will follow.

Baptist Medical Center, Columbia
Columbia, SC

Beth Israel Deaconess Medical Center
Boston, MA

Blue Cross and Blue Shield
of Massachusetts
Boston, MA

The Cambridge Hospital
Cambridge, MA

Cedars-Sinai Medical Center
Los Angeles, CA

Children's Hospital, Boston
Boston, MA

Children's Hospital of Philadelphia
Philadelphia, PA

Dana-Farber Cancer Institute
Boston, MA

Dartmouth-Hitchcock Medical Center
Lebanon, NH

Deaconess-Nashoba Hospital
Ayer, MA

Deaconess-Waltham Hospital
Waltham, MA

Fairview Health System
Minneapolis, MN

Kaiser Foundation Health Plan, Inc.
Oakland, CA

- Kaiser Permanente,
  Northern California Region
  Oakland, CA
- Kaiser Permanente,
  Southern California Region
  Anaheim, CA

Kaweah Delta Health Care District
Visalia, CA

Kimball Medical Center
Lakewood, NJ

Loss Prevention Foundation
Pontiac, MI

- Bay Medical Center
  Bay City, MI
- Garden City Hospital
  Garden City, MI
- Mt. Clemens General Hospital
  Mt. Clemens, MI
- Pontiac Osteopathic Hospital
  Medical Center
  Pontiac, MI

Lucile Salter Packard Children's Hospital at Stanford
Palo Alto, CA

Maine Medical Center
Portland, ME

Mercy Hospital
Miami, FL

Methodist Hospital/HealthSystem Minnesota
St. Louis Park, MN

Morton Plant Mease Health Care
Dunedin, FL

Munson Medical Center
Traverse City, MI

North Iowa Mercy Health Center
Mason City, IA

Northwest Covenant Medical Center
Denville, NJ

Paoli Memorial Hospital
Paoli, PA

Promina Gwinnett Health System
Lawrenceville, GA

SSM Health Care
St. Louis, MO

- Good Samaritan Regional Health Center
  Mount Vernon, IL
- St. Marys Hospital Medical Center
  Madison, WI

Suburban Hospital
Bethesda, MD

United Health Services Hospitals
Binghamton, NY

United Hospital/Allina Health System
St. Paul, MN

University of Chicago Hospitals and Health Systems
Chicago, IL

The Valley Hospital
Ridgewood, NJ

VHA East/New Jersey
Cranbury, NJ

- Elizabeth General Medical Center
  Elizabeth, NJ
- Grand View Hospital
  Sellersville, PA
- Lehigh Valley Hospital
  Allentown, PA

VHA Pennsylvania
Pittsburgh, PA

- Allegheny General Hospital
  Pittsburgh, PA
- Latrobe Area Hospital
  Latrobe, PA

Wesley Medical Center
Wichita, KS

PLANNING GROUP

The Institute for Healthcare Improvement thanks the Collaborative Chair and Director and the members of the Planning Group for dedicating their time and energy to teach and coach the Collaborative participants. Their generosity stems from a shared belief that much is known about how to reduce adverse drug events, and that applying that knowledge in a nonpunitive manner will ensure safer health care for millions of children and adults.

Collaborative Chair
Lucian L. Leape, MD
Adjunct Professor of Health Policy
Department of Health Policy and Management
Harvard School of Public Health
Boston, MA

Collaborative Director
Andrea Kabcenell, RN, MPH
Institute for Healthcare Improvement
Boston, MA

G. Ross Baker, PhD
Associate Professor
Department of Health Administration
University of Toronto
Toronto, ON, Canada

Michael R. Cohen, RPh, MS, FASHP
President
Institute for Safe Medication Practices
Warminster, PA

Frank Federico, RPh
Director of Pharmacy
Children's Hospital, Boston
Boston, MA

Donald Goldmann, MD
Hospital Epidemiologist
Medical Director of Quality Improvement
Children's Hospital, Boston
Boston, MA

Joseph Kasper, ScD, MBA
Adjunct Professor of Engineering
Adjunct Professor of Community and Family Medicine
Dartmouth College
Hanover, NH

Thomas W. Nolan, PhD
Statistician
Associates in Process Improvement
Silver Spring, MD

ADVISORS

In addition, the Institute for Healthcare Improvement thanks the following people for their valuable contributions to the Collaborative on Reducing Adverse Drug Events.

David Bates, MD, MSCI
Division of General Medicine and Primary Care
Brigham and Women's Hospital
Boston, MA

Marilyn Sue Bogner, PhD
President and Chief Scientist
Institute for the Study of Medical Error
Bethesda, MD

Robert L. Helmreich, PhD
Director
Aerospace Crew Research Project
Department of Psychology
University of Texas at Austin
Austin, TX

Charles E. Myers, MS, MBA
Director
Professional Practice and Scientific Affairs
American Society of Health-System Pharmacists
Bethesda, MD

Introduction The Challenge

Adverse drug events—injuries caused by the use (or nonuse) of a drug—affect as many as 1.5 million hospital patients annually, at a cost of three to four billion dollars. As many as half of these adverse drug events are caused by errors and are, therefore, preventable.

"The biggest challenge is to get people in hospitals—physicians, pharmacists, nurses, and administrators—to recognize that errors are systems problems and not people problems."

Lucian L. Leape, MD
Adjunct Professor of Health Policy
Department of Health Policy and Management
Harvard School of Public Health

"We need not tolerate current rates of error and hazard. But in pursuit of safety, 'trying harder' won't work. Improvement of safety in health care and the continuous reduction of error depend on the design and redesign of our systems of work."

Donald M. Berwick, MD
President and CEO, Institute for Healthcare Improvement

When errors occur, health care providers tend to look for an individual to blame. This punitive approach inhibits the reporting of errors. An unreported error cannot be investigated. Without investigation, the cause of the error goes undetected. Studies have shown that as many as 95% of medication errors go unreported. As a result, administrators are frequently unaware of the magnitude of the medication error problem, and therefore see little need to devote resources to correcting it.

Human factors specialists (cognitive psychologists and engineers who study human behavior) have shown that blame is misplaced when it focuses on the individual. Errors are rarely due to faulty people—almost no one errs on purpose. Most are caused by faulty systems that make errors both more likely to occur and more difficult to detect before they cause harm. Effective error prevention, therefore, requires redesigning systems.

"Unlike industry, which scrutinizes systems for error potential, the health care community often waits for accidents to occur before taking appropriate preventive action. This mentality perpetuates a serious health problem—adverse drug events. Working together, we can identify real and potential problems, seek workable solutions, and be proactive in our approach to providing safe patient care."

Michael Cohen, RPh, MS, FASHP
President, Institute for Safe Medication Practices

The Goal

In March 1996, 43 health care organizations began working together to reduce adverse drug events (ADEs) as part of the Institute for Healthcare Improvement's Breakthrough Series. Their goal: reduce ADEs by 30% or more within 12 months. This aggressive goal conveyed an important message: Small, incremental changes would not be enough; only significant, breakthrough changes would produce the desired results.

Figure 0.1

Increase in Time Between Medication Errors in the ICU

Baptist Medical Center, Columbia
Columbia, SC

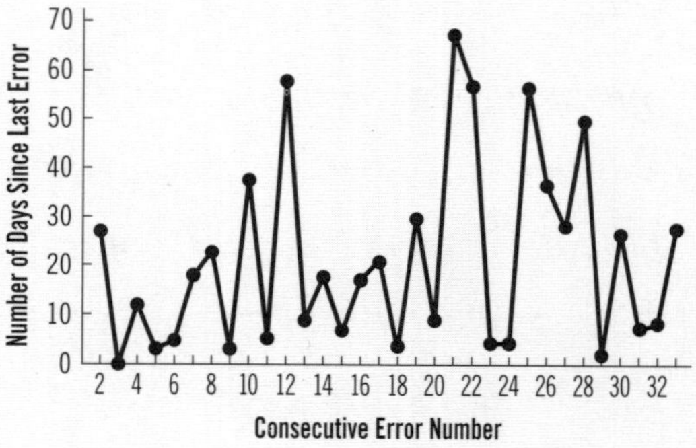

Because serious errors are rare events, some organizations find it useful to track the time between errors as an indication of whether changes in the medication system are leading to improvement (a longer duration indicates better results). In January 1996, the mean time between serious errors in the intensive care unit was 10 days. By January 1997, the mean time between serious errors increased to 20.8 days.

Figure 0.2

Reduction in Nonstandard or Illegible Orders

Munson Medical Center
Traverse City, MI

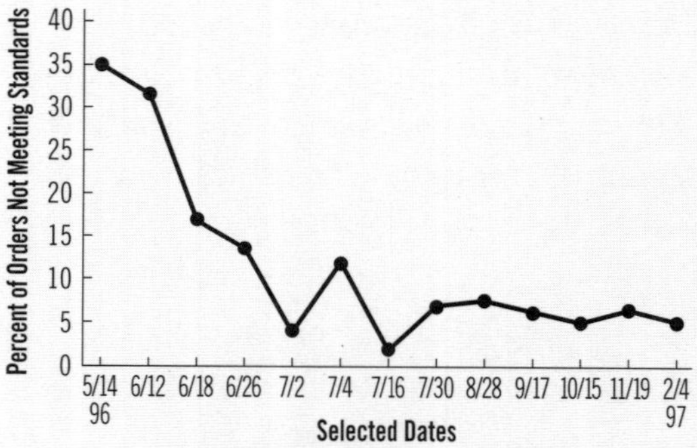

Average number of orders per day on one unit = 164

In May 1996, 35% of the orders monitored were either nonstandard—missing information or using incorrect abbreviations—or illegible. Such orders could be easily misunderstood or misread. Within nine months, the rate of nonstandard or illegible orders decreased to 5%.

The Results

Three-fourths of the organizations made notable progress in reducing ADEs and, of those, one-third met or exceeded their goal of 30% reduction in adverse drug events within 12 months. Others made substantial progress in understanding the error-prone parts of their medication systems and in improving their processes for ordering, dispensing, and administering medication. More importantly, most organizations are continuing to make new changes to reduce adverse drug events.

Figure 0.3
Improved Anticoagulation Control

Fairview Health System
Minneapolis, MN

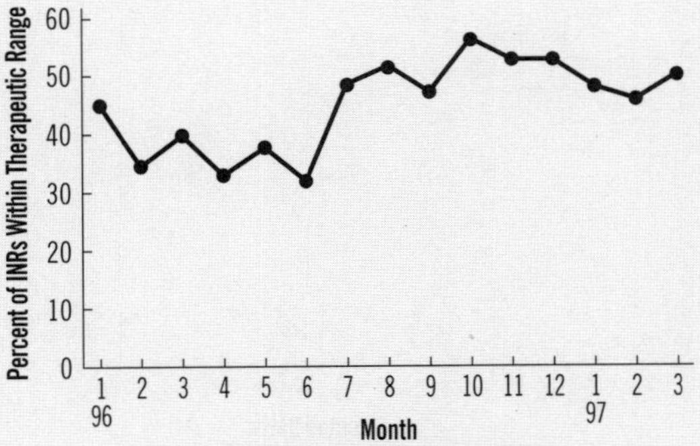

Average number of INRs drawn per month = 316

In January 1996, less than 45% of International Normalized Ratio (INR) test results for patients on warfarin were within therapeutic range. Within four months of establishing a warfarin clinic to assist with the outpatient management of anticoagulants, 58% of INRs drawn were within therapeutic range, and the new level remained stable for the next six months.

Figure 0.4
Increased On-time Medications

Methodist Hospital/HealthSystem Minnesota
St. Louis Park, MN

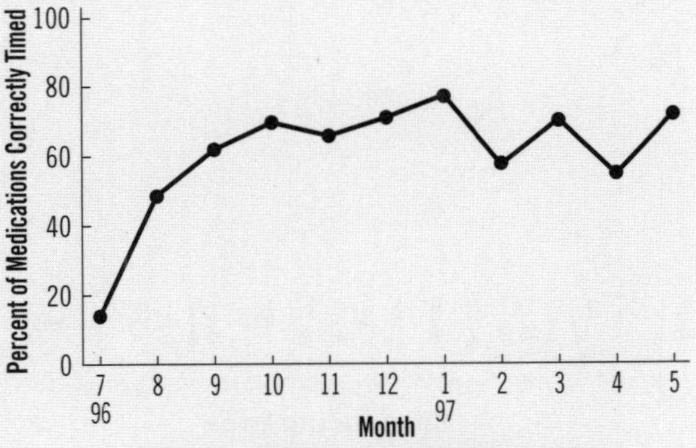

Average number of time-sensitive medication orders per month = 1,020 on a 49-bed unit

In July 1996, "time-sensitive" medications were scheduled for administration correctly only 14% of the time. Within six months, the accuracy of timing these medications had increased to 74%, and the new level remained stable at around 65%.

Part 1

A Model for Accelerating Improvement

This section introduces the model for accelerating improvement used by organizations in the Breakthrough Series. A case study shows how one organization used the model to reduce adverse drug events.

A Model for Accelerating Improvement

Organizations in the Breakthrough Series use a simple yet powerful model for accelerating improvement. The model is not meant to replace change models that organizations may already be using, but rather to accelerate improvement.

The model has two parts:

- Three fundamental questions, which can be addressed in any order.
- The Plan-Do-Study-Act (PDSA) cycle to test and implement changes in real work settings.

The Model for Improvement was initially developed by Thomas W. Nolan, PhD, and colleagues at Associates in Process Improvement, as a framework for accelerating improvement in a variety of business contexts (see Langley G, Nolan K, Nolan T, Norman C, Provost L. *The Improvement Guide: A Practical Approach to Enhancing Organizational Performance.* San Francisco: Jossey-Bass Publishers; 1996).

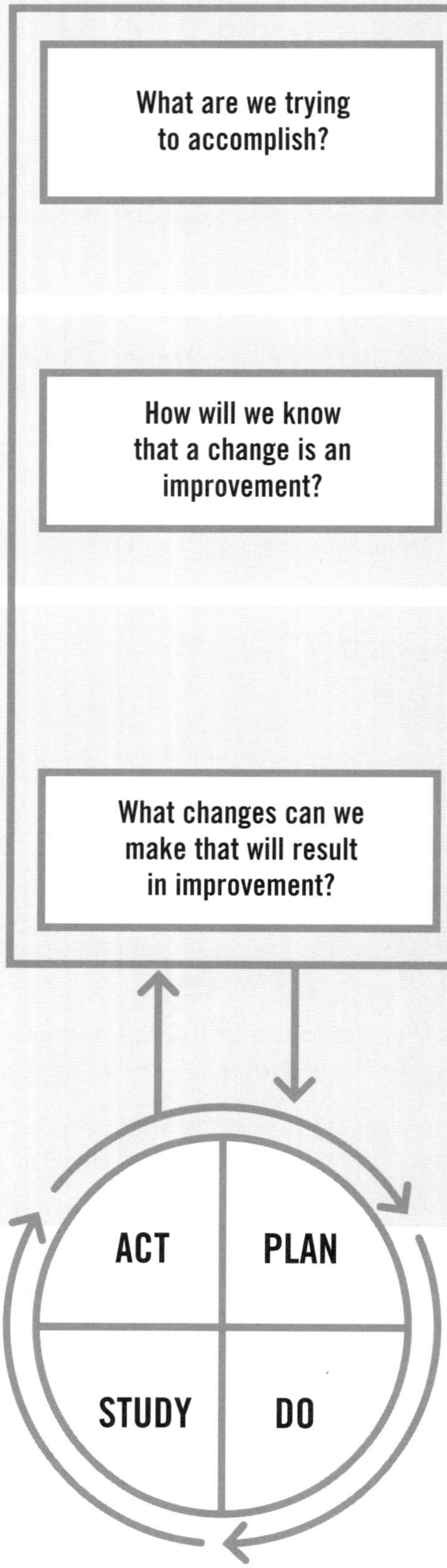

Setting Aims

Improvement requires setting aims. An organization will not improve without a clear and firm intention to do so. The aim should be expressed in specific terms—for example, 30% reduction in adverse drug events, 100% reduction in repeat hospitalizations for asthma, 30% reduction in cesarean section rates, 50% reduction in delays in surgery. Agreement on the aim is crucial. So is allocation of the people and resources necessary to accomplish the aim.

Establishing Measures

Measurement is an important part of the improvement process. Teams use quantitative measures to determine if a specific change actually leads to an improvement. Measures should provide information. For example, were dosing errors reduced? How many medications were given on time? How many doses were modified promptly in response to lab findings? How many nonstandard orders were intercepted in the pharmacy?

Developing Changes

All improvement requires making a change, but not all changes result in improvement. Organizations must, therefore, identify the changes that are most likely to result in improvement.

Ideas for change can come from a variety of sources: critical thinking about the current system, creative thinking, observing the process, a hunch, an innovation from another organization, an idea from the scientific literature, or an insight gleaned from a completely different situation. This Guide refers to good ideas for change as "change concepts." A change concept is a general idea—with proven merit and a sound scientific or logical foundation—that can stimulate specific ideas for changes that lead to improvement. Using change concepts and combining them creatively can inspire new ways of thinking about how to improve processes.

See Part 3, Change Concepts for Reducing Adverse Drug Events, for a comprehensive list of change concepts and specific ideas for changes generated from those concepts.

Change concepts lead to specific ideas for ways to improve a process. For example, a team may wish to simplify the process of administering narcotics. Using the change concept, "Simplify," the team might generate the following ideas for specific process changes:

- Reduce the number of dose strengths of morphine in stock.
- Use only one kind of patient controlled analgesia pump (PCA pump) on each nursing unit.
- Remove rarely used narcotics from the narcotics box.

In this way, a team can generate several process changes from a single change concept. The team then tests these changes to see if they lead to improvement.

Once a team has set an aim, established measures to indicate whether a change leads to an improvement, and found a promising idea for change, the next step is to test that change in the real work setting by conducting a Plan-Do-Study-Act (PDSA) cycle.

For an example of how to document a PDSA cycle, see the Improvement Cycle Worksheet in Part 6, Resources for Reducing Adverse Drug Events.

Testing Changes

THE PLAN-DO-STUDY-ACT (PDSA) CYCLE

The Model for Improvement is based on a trial-and-learning approach to improvement. The PDSA cycle is shorthand for testing a change—by trying it, observing the consequences, and then learning from those consequences.

Teams need to address several challenges in each step of the PDSA cycle:

Step 1 Plan

- State the objective of the cycle.
- Make predictions about what will happen and why.
- Develop a plan to test the change. (Who? What? When? Where? What data need to be collected?)

Step 2 Do

- Carry out the test.
- Document problems and unexpected observations.
- Begin analysis of the data.

Step 3 Study

- Complete the analysis of the data.
- Compare the data to the predictions.
- Summarize what was learned.

Step 4 Act

- Determine what modifications should be made.
- Prepare a plan for the next cycle.

FYI

"What can we do by next Tuesday?"

Organizations that want to improve should begin small-scale tests of change as soon as possible. Running small-scale cycles soon works far better than running large-scale cycles after a long period of planning.

Even an ambitious and innovative change should be tested first on a small scale—for example, with only one or two attending physicians or with the next three diabetic patients. Each PDSA cycle, properly done, provides valuable information and forms the basis for further improvement. If a change works on a small scale and is improved in successive PDSA cycles, it can then be implemented with assurance on a larger scale.

LINKING PLAN-DO-STUDY-ACT CYCLES

The completion of each PDSA cycle leads directly into the start of the next cycle. A team learns from the test (What worked and what didn't work? What should be kept, changed, or abandoned?) and uses the new knowledge to plan the next test. The team continues linking PDSA cycles in this way, refining the change until it is ready for broader implementation.

People are far more willing to test a change when they know that changes can and will be modified as needed. Linking small cycles helps overcome an organization's natural resistance to change.

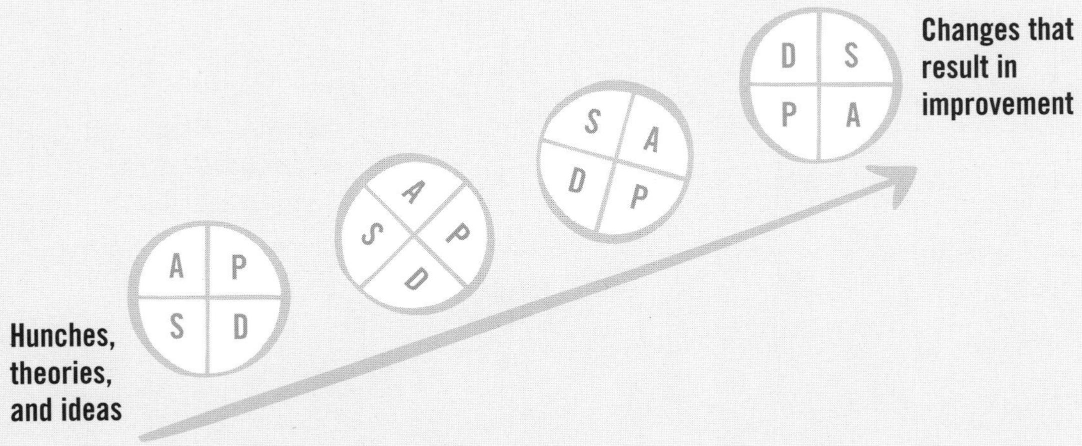

SEVERAL LINKED CYCLES

Often, teams test more than one change at a time, each aimed at achieving the same ultimate goal.

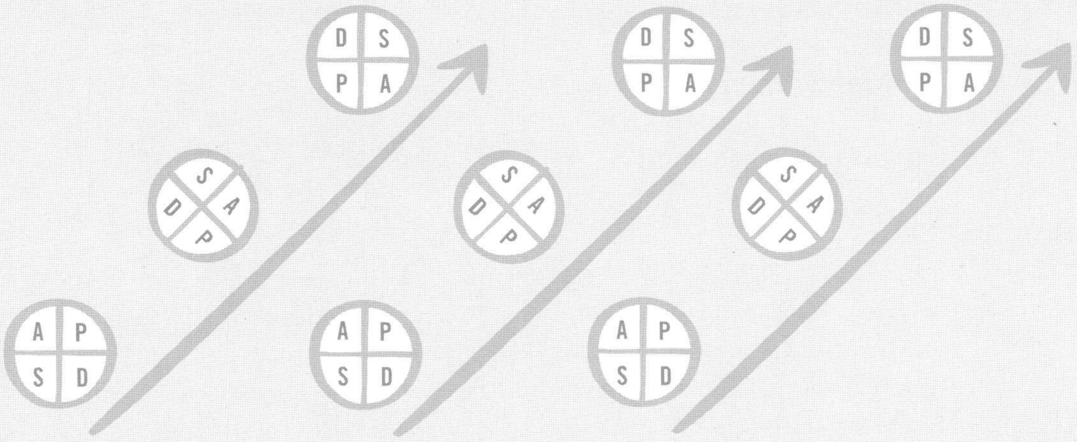

Case Study Fairview Health System

Fairview Health System in Minneapolis, MN, is an integrated system consisting of four community hospitals, one university teaching hospital, four nursing homes, a home health agency, 3,000 community-based primary and specialty care physicians, 5,000 employees, and other service providers.

The system's leadership, recognizing that there were multiple opportunities for error in the hospitals within the system, set out to minimize the risk of error by restructuring the medication system.

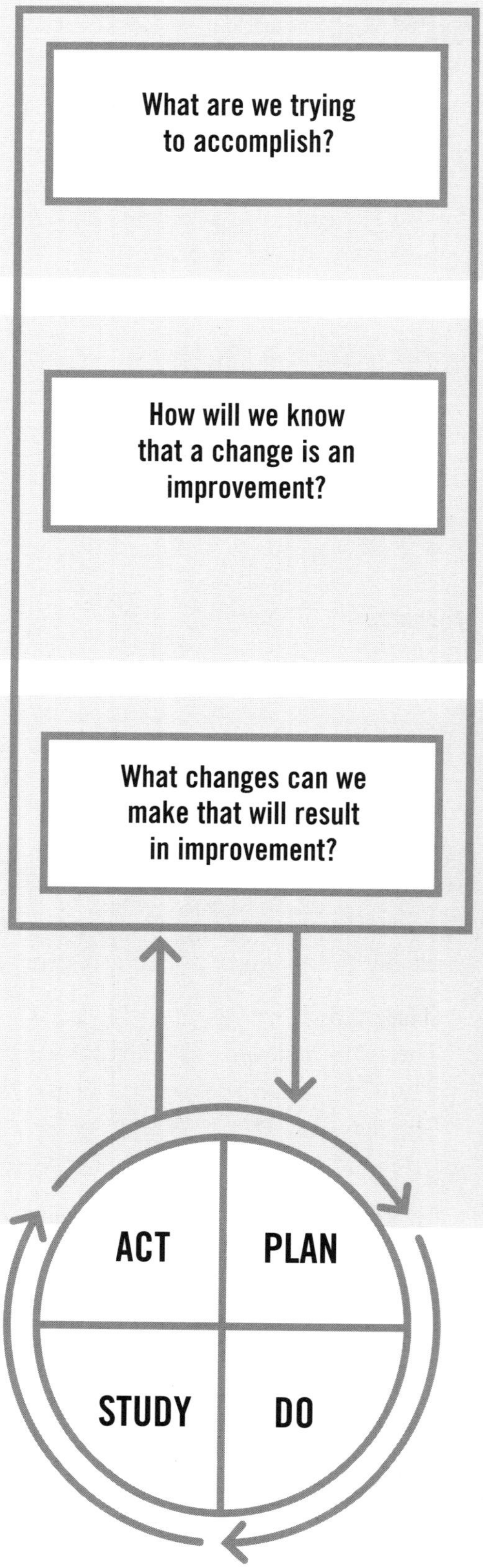

Setting Aims

The team set the following aim:

Reduce to zero potential adverse drug events in the ordering, dispensing, and administration of chemotherapy, insulin, warfarin, and hypnotics.

A *potential adverse drug event (PADE)* is a serious medication error that had the potential to cause harm to the patient but, either by luck or interception, did not.

Establishing Measures

The team established the following measure for improvement for each process in the medication system—ordering, dispensing, and administration: A change is an improvement if the number of PADEs per order or per patient decreases. The pharmacist counted the number of PADEs per order in each area—chemotherapy, insulin, warfarin, and hypnotics—during the review of the physician's order prior to dispensing the drug.

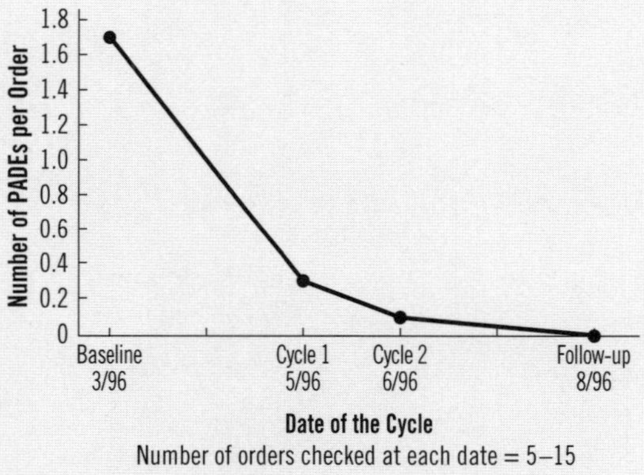

Figure 1.1
Reduction in Potential Adverse Drug Events (PADEs) per Order

Fairview Health System
Minneapolis, MN

Developing Changes

In order to identify the most promising ideas for specific changes, the team began with the following two change concepts:

- **Standardize**
  The team believed that if physicians wrote orders using standard forms, variation would decrease and, consequently, there would be fewer opportunities for error. The team decided to develop standard chemotherapy order forms and to standardize the maximum dose for each medication.
- **Use Constraints and Forcing Functions**
  The team looked for ways to use forcing functions to error-proof the medication system. The team decided to institute automatic drug substitution for specific drugs such as hypnotics and antihistamines, and automatic dose reduction in the pharmacy for a variety of drugs for patients with renal dysfunction. In addition, the team decided to remove high-hazard drugs from the formulary and from the floor stock.

See Part 3, Change Concepts for Reducing Adverse Drug Events, for an explanation of these change concepts.

Testing Changes

CHANGE 1: Standardize chemotherapy ordering and dispensing.

The team believed that standardizing practices would enhance communication and reduce variation in the ordering, dispensing, and administration of chemotherapy.

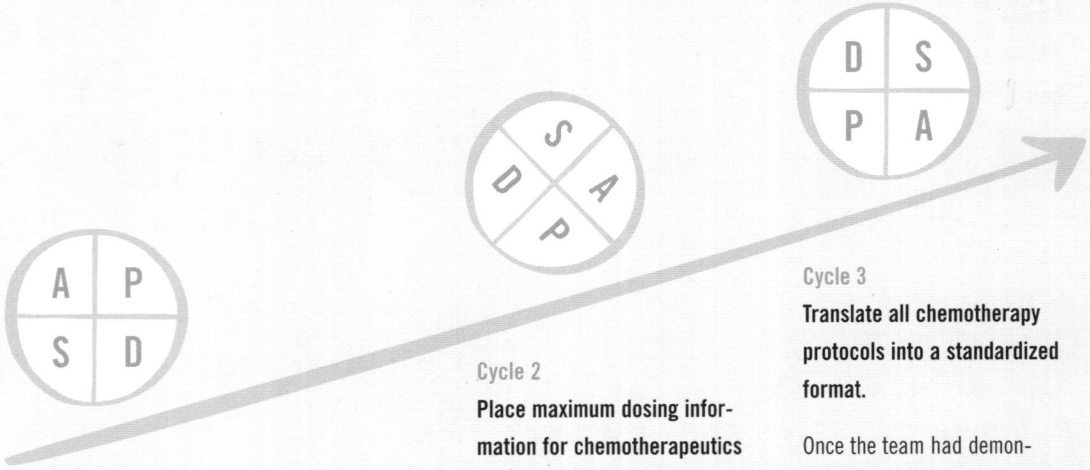

Cycle 1

Devise a standard preprinted chemotherapy order form.

Using preprinted forms ensures that the ordering physician will include key demographic data as well as required information about the drug. Forms help to clarify and define responsibilities in the chemotherapy medication process and to guide choices such as method of administration, administration dates, and frequency. They also allow a triple check of calculations.

See Part 4, Achieving Breakthrough Improvement in Reducing Adverse Drug Events, pp. 124–125, for an example of a preprinted chemotherapy order form.

Cycle 2

Place maximum dosing information for chemotherapeutics on a chart that is available to all clinicians.

Cycle 3

Translate all chemotherapy protocols into a standardized format.

Once the team had demonstrated the efficacy of standardization, it made sure that all chemotherapy protocols were available in a standardized, easy-to-use format.

Process Measure

The pharmacy measured the number of PADEs per chemotherapy order and classified them by their stage in the process—clarification, transcription, or information. The team measured PADEs at four different times:

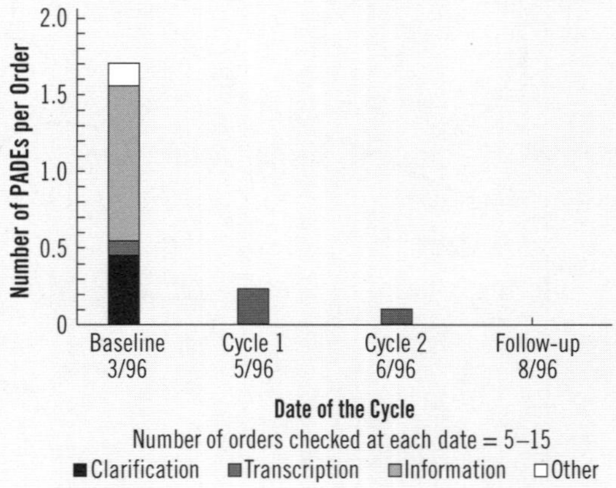

Figure 1.2

Reduction in Potential Adverse Drug Events per Order, Classified by Location of Error

Fairview Health System
Minneapolis, MN

- Before the standardization process began (Baseline)
- At two points during the testing process (Cycle 1 and Cycle 2)
- One month after the changes were complete (Follow-up)

In just five months, the number of measured PADEs per order fell from 1.7 to zero.

CHANGE 2: Establish automatic dosing protocols to prevent toxic doses.

Certain medications must be dosed individually, according to patient status. However, pertinent information about the patient's status may not be available or may not come to the attention of the ordering physician. Setting up an automatic dosing system in the pharmacy is a way to ensure appropriate dosing changes.

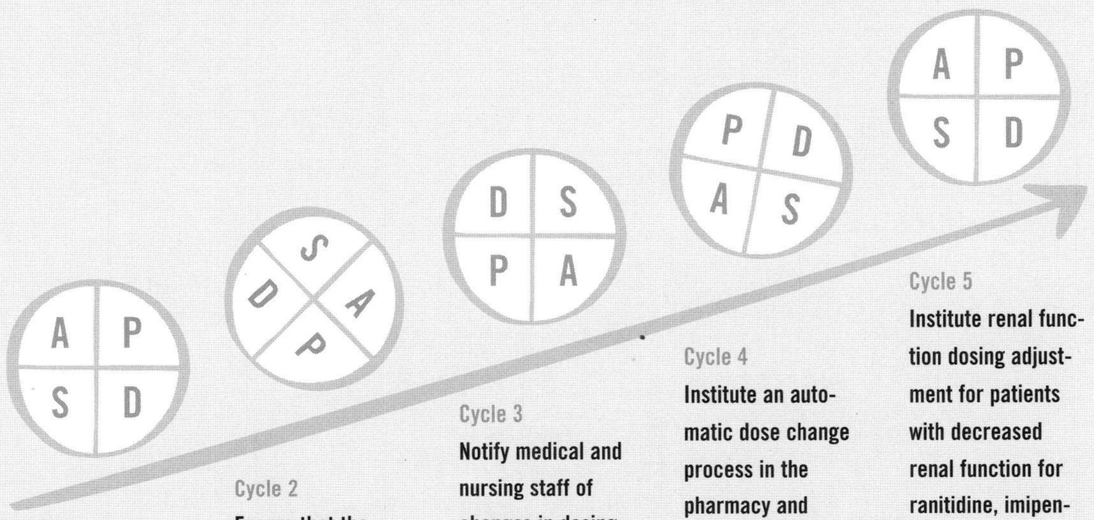

Cycle 1
Identify medications that require dosing modification based on patient status.

Cycle 2
Ensure that the pharmacy has information on patient age, height, weight, and renal function.

Cycle 3
Notify medical and nursing staff of changes in dosing.

Cycle 4
Institute an automatic dose change process in the pharmacy and rewrite pretyped orders to account prospectively for age-related dosing.

Cycle 5
Institute renal function dosing adjustment for patients with decreased renal function for ranitidine, imipenem, allopurinol, B-lactam antibiotics, and co-trimoxazole. Institute automatic reduction for doses of hypnotic medications for patients over 65 years old.

Process Measure

The team measured the percentage of benzodiazepine orders for patients over 65 that were filled with the correct doses and the percentage filled with doses that were correct for age.

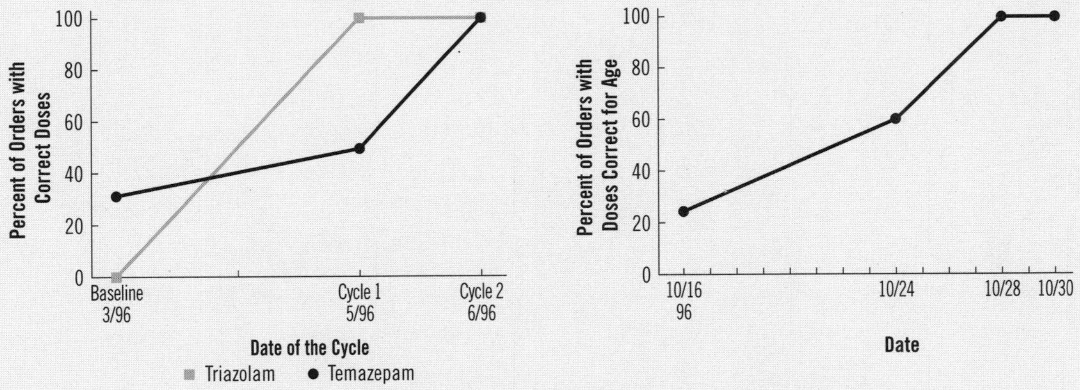

Number of doses checked at each date = 6–10

Figure 1.3
Benzodiazepine Orders for Patients over 65
- **Increase in Correct Doses**
- **Increase in Doses Correct for Age**

Fairview Health System
Minneapolis, MN

CHANGE 3: Remove dangerous drugs from the formulary.

Certain medications are known to be hazardous for specific conditions or in interaction with certain food and drugs. They are used only if the benefits outweigh the risks. Eliminating the more dangerous drugs will reduce potential adverse drug events when safer drugs that serve the same purpose are available.

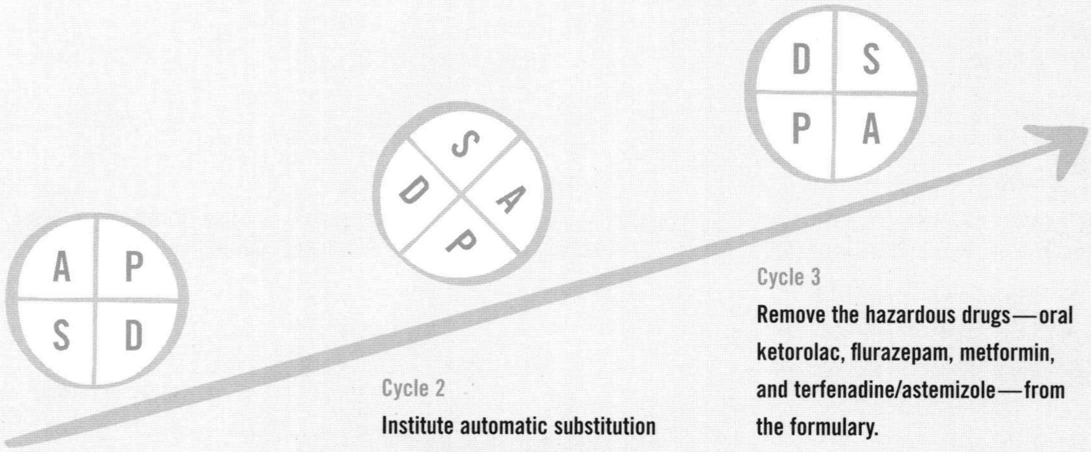

Cycle 1

Identify drugs in the formulary constituting an unnecessary risk—that is, hazardous drugs for which a safer substitute is available.

Cycle 2

Institute automatic substitution of safer drugs when one of these hazardous drugs is ordered. Notify staff of these changes and the substitution protocol.

Cycle 3

Remove the hazardous drugs—oral ketorolac, flurazepam, metformin, and terfenadine/astemizole—from the formulary.

Figure 1.4
Dangerous Drugs Removed from the Formulary

Fairview Health System
Minneapolis, MN

Medication	Doses per year avoided
oral ketorolac	1,700 doses
flurazepam	1,500 doses
metformin	2,000 doses
terfenadine/astemizole	1,700 doses

CHANGE 4: Remove hazardous drugs from the ICU floor stock.

Certain drugs are hazardous but necessary. Removing these drugs from the floor stock and providing them premixed when needed decreases the risk of misuse. The team removed vials of dopamine, dobutamine, IV nitroglycerin, potassium chloride, NPH and Lente insulin, and heparin 10,000-unit/500 mL and 25,000-unit/500 mL bags from the floor stock. Now the pharmacy either mixes these or supplies a stock of premixed infusions (excluding heparin) to the unit.

Results

BREAKTHROUGH IMPROVEMENT

By making specific changes based on the change concepts, "Standardize" and "Use Constraints and Forcing Functions," Fairview Health System reduced potential adverse drug events to near zero in several areas:

- **chemotherapy ordering**
- **adverse events from specific drugs**
- **administration of concentrated doses of specific drugs**

In addition, Fairview achieved appropriate benzodiazepine dosing in 100% of patients over 65 years of age.

THUS FAR IN THE GUIDE, YOU HAVE LEARNED:

Part 1 *The Model for Improvement, which can be applied to any area you want to improve.*

Part 2

A Step-by-Step Guide to Reducing Adverse Drug Events

In this section, you'll learn how to begin working on reducing adverse drug events in your organization. Each step—setting aims, forming the team, establishing measures, and developing and testing changes—is illustrated with examples showing how organizations have used the Model for Improvement to bring about significant reductions in adverse drug events in a short period of time.

Setting Aims

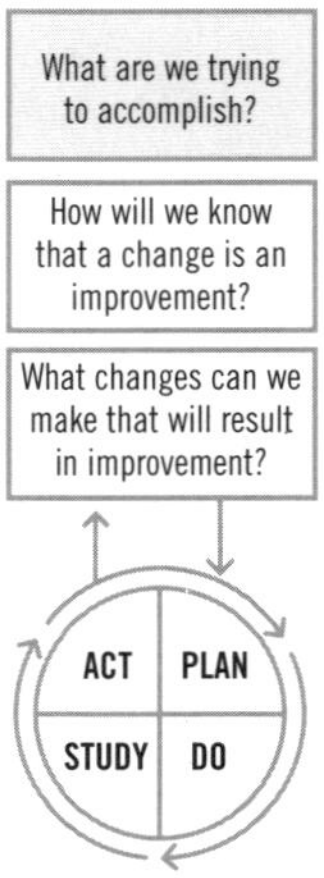

Improvement requires setting aims. A clearly stated, mutually agreed-upon aim will help teams stay on track throughout their improvement efforts.

PRINCIPLES OF AN EFFECTIVE AIM STATEMENT

1. State the aim clearly.

Achieving agreement on the aim of a project is critical for maintaining progress. Teams make better progress when they are very specific about their aims.

2. Include numerical goals.

Including numerical goals clarifies expectations. Are small, incremental improvements expected, or are large, breakthrough changes necessary? For example, the aim stated as "Reduce adverse drug events" does not communicate expectations as clearly as "Reduce adverse drug events in critical care by 30% within 12 months." Including a numerical goal and a time frame also helps team members begin to think about what their measures of improvement will be, what initial changes they might make, and what level of support they will need.

3. Set stretch goals.

Setting stretch goals—for example, "Reduce adverse drug events in critical care by 30% within 12 months"—communicates immediately and clearly that maintaining the *status quo* is not an option. Effective leaders communicate both the feasibility of goals and the need to do more than tweak the existing system to meet those goals. Once this is clear, people begin to look for ways to overcome barriers to achieving the stretch goals.

4. Avoid aim drift.

Once the aim has been set, the team needs to be careful not to back away from it. The initial stretch goal—"Reduce adverse drug events in critical care by 30% within 12 months"—can slip almost imperceptibly to "Reduce adverse drug events by 15%" or "by 10%." To avoid aim drift, repeat the aim continually. Start each team meeting with an explicit statement of aim, for example, "Remember, we're here to reduce our ADE rate in critical care by 30% within the next 12 months," and then review progress quantitatively over time.

5. Be prepared to refocus the aim.

Every team needs to recognize when to refocus its aim. If the team's overall aim is system level (for example, "Reduce adverse drug events in critical care by 30% within 12 months"), the team members may find that focusing for a time on a smaller part of the system (for example, "Reduce adverse drug events *for critical care patients on the cardiac service* by 30% within 12 months") will help them achieve the desired system-level goal. *Note:* Don't confuse aim drift, or backing away from a stretch goal (which usually isn't a good tactic), with consciously deciding to work on a smaller part of the system (which often is a good tactic).

1 Baptist Medical Center, Columbia Columbia, SC

Background: Baptist Medical Center is a 524-bed, private, not-for-profit, acute care hospital located in downtown Columbia. The hospital provides inpatient and outpatient services and treats nearly 44,000 patients in its emergency department each year. The intensive care unit has 18 beds and provides both medical and surgical services. While the ICU had reported no particular problems with medication errors, the team decided to focus on this high-hazard area because of its fast pace, the high volume of drugs used, and the critical status of its patients.

2 Lucile Salter Packard Children's Hospital at Stanford Palo Alto, CA

Background: Packard Children's Hospital is a 206-bed acute care teaching hospital affiliated with Stanford Medical Center. The team began with a very broad aim—reduce medication errors in the hospital by 50% in 12 months—but soon found that it needed to narrow the aim in order to focus its improvement efforts.

Examples of Effective Aim Statements

1 — Aim:
Reduce medication errors in the ICU by 25% within 12 months.

The team believed that this was a stretch goal—challenging, but not unattainable.

2 — Aim:
Reduce medication errors in the entire hospital by reaching the following goals within 12 months:

- Eliminate cardiovascular drip errors in the neonatal intensive care unit (NICU).
- Decrease physician prescribing errors by 20%.
- Decrease errors in chemotherapy administration by 20%.

These goals focused the team's efforts on improving three specific areas, each of great concern. Improvements in these areas would help reduce errors housewide. The first goal—eliminating cardiovascular drip errors—was a stretch goal, but one that the team felt was important. Variation in practice around this critical process and reports of near misses convinced the team to take on this challenging goal.

AIM

3 Pontiac Osteopathic Hospital Medical Center Pontiac, MI

Background: Pontiac Osteopathic is a 296-bed urban acute care hospital. It is a member of the Loss Prevention Foundation, a malpractice risk cooperative. In 1995, the Loss Prevention Foundation noted an increase in medication incidents in one of its member hospitals. The Foundation elected to enroll as a group in the Breakthrough Series Collaborative, with four of its member hospitals sending a representative. The team from Pontiac Osteopathic Hospital was concerned about medication errors hospital-wide, but elected to initiate changes in one particular unit.

Aim:
Reduce adverse drug events in the cardiac monitoring unit (CMU) by 50% within 12 months.

This aim is specific with respect to the location, the level of change desired, and the time frame for improvement. This specificity helped focus the team's efforts and prevent distractions. The goal of 50% reduction was ambitious but not out of reach; it signaled that the status quo was not an option.

4 Promina Gwinnett Health System Lawrenceville, GA

Background: The Promina Gwinnett Health System is a not-for-profit health care network in metropolitan Atlanta. The system has five facilities with a total of 390 licensed beds. The team began with the broad aim of reducing adverse drug events by 40%. The team then decided on four areas of focus and developed an aim for each. The following is one of those four aims.

Aim:
Reduce errors in the medication ordering and administration processes by 20% within 12 months.

The team specified three strategies for meeting the aim:

- Improve the ordering and administration of heparin.
- Decrease illegible and nonstandard orders.
- Standardize routine orders.

Because 22% of all the serious errors involved heparin, a potentially lethal drug, the team began by working on improving heparin ordering and administration.

Forming the Team

Getting the right people on the team is critical to a successful improvement effort. Teams vary in size and composition; each organization builds teams to suit its own needs. Teams working on reducing adverse drug events should include members familiar with the different parts of the medication system—managers and administrators, as well as those who work daily in the process, such as physicians, pharmacists, and nurses.

A team's composition depends on its aim:

First, review the aim.

Second, consider the system that relates to that aim: What processes will be affected by the improvement?

Third, be sure that the team includes individuals who can drive improvement in those areas.

Team members should be able to meet relatively frequently, work efficiently, and test changes quickly. Perhaps the most important single success factor for a team is commitment to working together toward a shared goal.

THREE INGREDIENTS OF AN EFFECTIVE TEAM

Effective teams have representation from three different kinds of expertise within the organization: system leadership, technical expertise, and day-to-day leadership. There may be one or more individuals on the team with each kind of expertise, or one individual may have expertise in more than one area, but all three areas should be represented in order to drive change.

System Leadership

SL

Teams need someone with enough authority in the organization to institute a change when one is suggested and to overcome barriers when they arise. The team's system leader understands the implications of proposed changes for various parts of the system. It is important that this person have authority in all areas that are affected by the change, including the authority to allocate the time and resources needed by the team to achieve its aim.

Technical Expertise

TE

Teams need subject matter experts, individuals who understand the scientific and technical foundations of the processes of care that are being improved. Additional technical support may also come from an expert on improvement methods, who can help a team understand what to measure, how to design tests of change, how to collect and display data, and how to understand and interpret the data.

Day-to-Day Leadership

DL

Teams also need someone who works on a daily basis in the process that is being improved and thus understands the process thoroughly. This person should understand or know how to find out the effects of any planned changes. This person should also have the desire and ability to drive the improvement project on a daily basis.

Examples of Effective Teams

1 Baptist Medical Center, Columbia
Columbia, SC

Aim: Reduce medication errors in the ICU by 25% within 12 months.

Team:

- SL Chair of the Pharmacy and Therapeutics Committee
- TE DL Clinical pharmacist
- DL Clinical nurse specialist from nursing support services
- TE Clinical nurse specialist from the ICU
- SL Assistant Director of Pharmacy
- Risk manager
- Nurse from perioperative services

In support of the team:

Vice President of Medical Affairs
Vice President of Administration/Nursing Services
Vice President of Administration/Pharmacy Services

This team began its work without significant system leadership in the ICU. It took some time to involve the ICU staff; initially, the clinical pharmacist and the clinical nurse specialist from nursing support services provided day-to-day team leadership. However, the team made rapid progress only after the ICU's clinical nurse specialist assumed more day-to-day leadership.

2 Lucile Salter Packard Children's Hospital at Stanford
Palo Alto, CA

Aim: Eliminate cardiovascular drip errors in the neonatal intensive care unit (NICU) within 12 months.

Team:

- Cardiovascular surgeon
- TE Anesthesiologist
- Neonatologist
- TE Clinical nurse specialist
- Staff nurse in the NICU
- DL Staff nurse in perioperative nursing
- Clinical pharmacist
- TE Quality management coordinator

In support of the team:

SL Vice President, Patient Care Services

Because this team was so focused on details of patient care, it was unable to get the needed system leadership on the team. Fortunately, because the culture at this hospital encouraged interdepartmental cooperation around improving clinical processes, the team was able to obtain the necessary resources without having a system leader as a regular member of the team.

TEAM

3 Pontiac Osteopathic Hospital Medical Center Pontiac, MI

Aim: Reduce adverse drug events in the cardiac monitoring unit (CMU) by 50% within 12 months.

Team:

- SL Director of Nursing
- SL Chief Executive Officer
- TE Director of Pharmacy
- TE DL Physician Director of Quality
- Attending physician who admits on the CMU
- CMU staff nurse
- Staff pharmacist

Initially, this team included many high-level managers. Early in its work, the team identified the need for additional staff familiar with local work processes. The team added staff nurses, staff pharmacists, and an attending physician. The senior leaders then took a less active role, but continued to support and monitor the work. The physician quality director drove the process, but staff members led implementation of changes.

4 Promina Gwinnett Health System Lawrenceville, GA

Aim: Reduce errors in the medication ordering and administration processes by 20% within 12 months.

Intermediate Aim: Improve the ordering and administration of heparin.

Team:

- DL Director of Nursing Quality Improvement
- SL TE Vice President, Systems Clinical Services
- SL TE Director of Pharmacy
- Clinical pharmacist

Forming a small team composed of senior leaders provides benefits and poses special challenges. System leadership is always available, but team members have many other demands on their time. In this team, the members switched roles so often that, at any time, one of them could take over the day-to day-leadership. All of the team members had technical expertise, but they enlisted the help of additional staff to implement changes. They did this on an ad hoc basis, depending on which part of the medication ordering process they were working on.

Establishing Measures

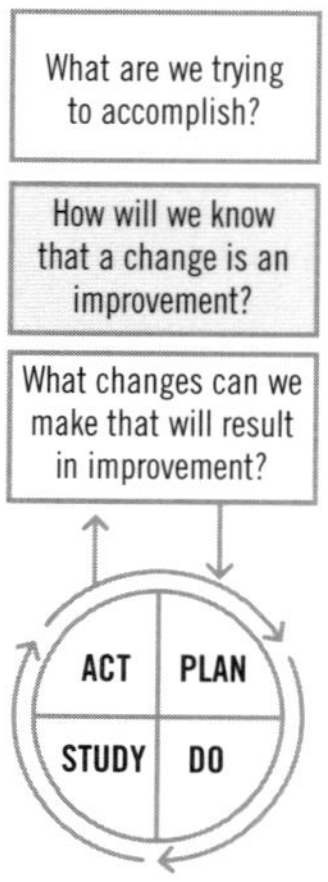

After setting a clear aim and forming the right team, the next step is establishing simple measures that will indicate if a change leads to an improvement. If a team has done a good job articulating its aim, it can easily define simple, effective measures.

Teams usually need to track both outcome and process measures:

Outcome measures tell a team whether changes are actually leading to improvement—that is, helping to achieve the stated aim.

- An example of an outcome measure is "reduction in errors due to misreading physician orders."

Process measures tell a team whether a specific process change has been accomplished and whether it is having the intended effect on the flow of work. A team often establishes several process measures in the course of its work, assuming that improvement in a process measure will eventually impact the outcome measure.

- An example of a process measure is "the percentage of medication orders that must be clarified because of illegibility."

See Six Methods for Measuring Errors in Health Care, pp. 40–47, at the end of Part 2.

Measurement should be used to speed change up, not to slow it down. Many organizations become bogged down in measurement, delaying making a change until they have collected enough data. The following tips can help teams use measurement to accelerate improvement.

TIPS FOR EFFECTIVE MEASUREMENT

1. Seek usefulness, not perfection.

Remember, measurement is not the goal; improvement is the goal. In order to move forward to the next step, a team needs just enough data to know whether changes are leading to improvement.

2. Use sampling.

Sampling is a simple, powerful way to help a team understand how a system is working. Instead of measuring all of something, measure a sample—every tenth order, or the next five patients, or ten randomly selected doses.

3. Plot data over time.

Improvement requires change, and change is, by definition, a temporal phenomenon. Much information about a system and how to improve it can be obtained by plotting data over time (for example, tracking the number of orders requiring pharmacy intervention over several weeks), indicating the points at which changes were made, and observing trends and other patterns.

4. Use a balanced set of measures.

Teams use "balancing measures" to make sure that changes designed to improve one part of the system aren't causing new problems in other parts of the system. For example, if a team has concentrated potassium chloride removed from the floor stock and mixed in the pharmacy, it needs to make sure that this change does not cause delays in the administration of emergency medications. Monitoring these potential ripple effects is essential.

5. Don't wait for the information system.

Much useful information already exists and can be obtained with relative ease. Don't wait for two months to receive the next quarter's incident reports or for two weeks to receive laboratory summaries. Use pencil and paper and collect the data this week.

6. Use qualitative and quantitative data.

For example, rather than delay testing a change until the data collection about errors is complete, ask three nurses, "What are the errors waiting to happen on this unit?" These qualitative judgments can be verified and data can be collected during tests of change.

7. Use outcome and process measures.

For example, if the aim is to decrease timing errors for preoperative antibiotics, the outcome measure is the percentage of antibiotics given on time. A process measure would be the percentage of patients who came to the operating room with the antibiotic dose the anesthesiologist will give taped to their charts.

1 Baptist Medical Center, Columbia Columbia, SC

Aim: Reduce medication errors in the ICU by 25% within 12 months.

2 Lucile Salter Packard Children's Hospital at Stanford Palo Alto, CA

Aim: Eliminate cardiovascular drip errors in the neonatal intensive care unit (NICU) within 12 months.

Examples of Effective Measures

1 Outcome Measure:

The time between medication errors in the ICU (longer is better).

Figure 2.1

Time Between Errors in the ICU

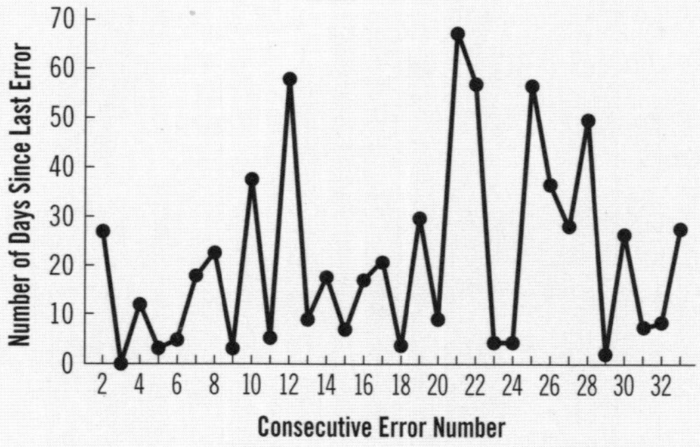

See Six Methods for Measuring Errors in Health Care, pp. 40–47, at the end of Part 2.

Changes to improve the medication process in the ICU yielded an increase in the time between serious errors, as measured by reported medication incidents. Measuring "days between errors" proved a useful way to track progress on rare events like serious medication errors. Assuming the reporting is reliable, an increase in the interval between errors indicates that the process improvements are leading to fewer errors.

2 Outcome Measure:

The percentage of NICU cardiovascular intravenous (IV) drips that were within the recommended therapeutic range.

Figure 2.2

Cardiovascular IV Drips for Selected Patients

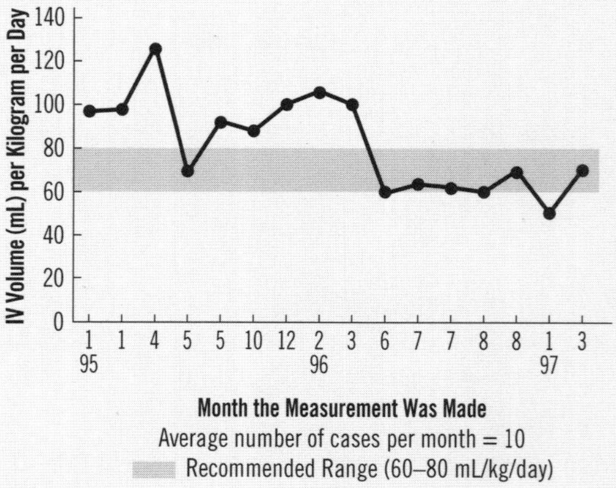

In the NICU, fluid volume overload indicates poorly managed IV solutions. This team decided to track the total volume infused to see if the changes they made helped keep cardiovascular IV drips within the recommended range. When the protocol was implemented, the volume infused fell into the recommended range.

Process Measures:

The team collected other types of information, including the number of cardiovascular drips that were appropriately labeled and the number of drips that needed to be changed within 48 hours of surgery.

3 Pontiac Osteopathic Hospital Medical Center Pontiac, MI

Aim: Reduce adverse drug events in the cardiac monitoring unit (CMU) by 50% within 12 months.

Outcome measure:

Errors per month in the cardiac monitoring unit.

Figure 2.3

Errors in the Cardiac Monitoring Unit

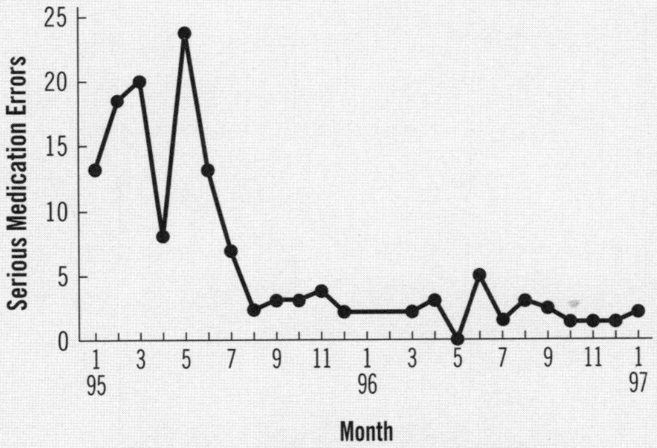

Average number of CMU patients per month = 333

This team tracked the errors per month in the cardiac monitoring unit over time, noting when specific changes were put into place. The team used sampling, reviewing a subset of charts every week rather than reviewing all charts, to monitor the process to see if the changes resulted in improvement.

4 Promina Gwinnett Health System Lawrenceville, GA

Aim: Reduce errors in the medication ordering and administration processes by 20% within 12 months.

Intermediate Aim: Improve the ordering and administration of heparin.

Outcome Measure:

The time to reach therapeutic aPTT.

Figure 2.4

Time to Reach Therapeutic aPTT

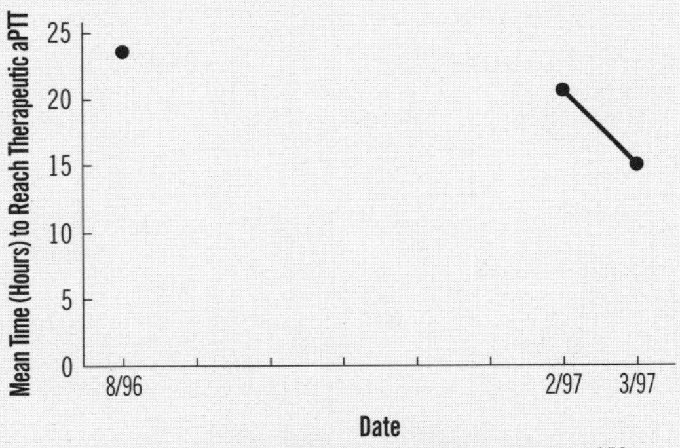

Average number of patients on heparin per month = 150

The team's aim was to improve the process for ordering and titrating heparin so that the patient safely reaches a therapeutic level of anticoagulation as soon as possible. Complexities in the ordering and administration processes impede appropriate anticoagulation. The team chose "time to reach a therapeutic blood level" as the measure for success. They set as a standard "reaching therapeutic range within 24 hours of initiating heparin therapy" and tracked the percentage of patients whose treatment met that standard.

Developing and Testing Changes

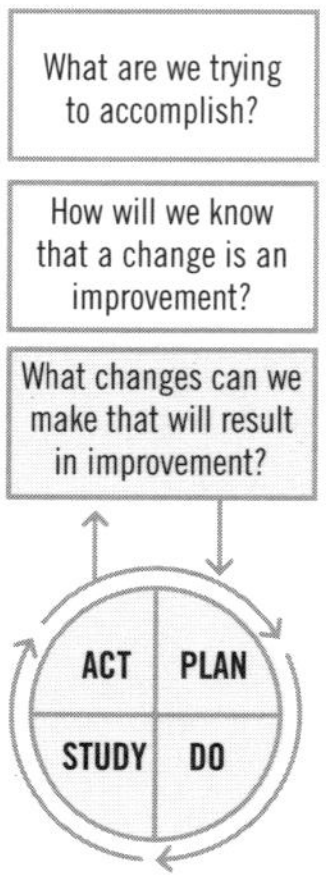

After setting a clear aim, forming the right team, and establishing simple measures to indicate if a change leads to an improvement, the next step is developing and testing changes.

TIPS FOR SUCCESSFUL TESTS OF CHANGE

1. Stay a cycle ahead.

When designing a test, imagine at the start what the subsequent test or two might be, given the various possible findings in the Study phase of the Plan-Do-Study-Act cycle.

2. Scale down the scope of tests.

Variables that can be scaled down include the following:

- The number of patients, doctors, and others involved in the test ("Sample the next 10" instead of "Get a sample of 200")
- The number of locations or amount of time involved in the test ("Test it on 5 West" or "Test it this week for patients on heparin" instead of "Test it in all clinics")

3. Pick willing volunteers.

Work with those who want to work with you. ("I know Dr. Jones will help us" instead of "How can we convince Dr. Smith to buy in?")

4. Avoid the need for consensus, buy-in, or political solutions.

Save these for later stages. When possible, choose changes that do not require long processes of approval from, for example, the Pharmacy and Therapeutics Committee.

5. Don't reinvent the wheel.

Instead, replicate changes made elsewhere. For example, use another organization's insulin sliding-dose scale. Assume that medications associated with errors in other hospitals are probably culprits in yours, as well.

6. Pick easy changes to try.

Look for the concepts that seem the most feasible and will have the greatest impact.

7. Avoid technical slowdowns.

Don't wait for the new computer to arrive; try paper and pencil instead.

8. Reflect on the results of every change.

Often, the "Study" phase is postponed or omitted, leaving the team with no information to guide next steps. Teams learn important lessons from successful and not-so-successful tests of change.

9. Be prepared to end test of a change.

If the test shows that a change or series of changes is not leading to improvement, it should be stopped. Successful teams find that they can learn just as much (or more) from "failed" tests of change as from "successful" tests. In this sense, the only real failure from a test of change is the failure to embrace it, reflect on it, and learn from it.

1 Baptist Medical Center, Columbia
Columbia, SC

Aim: Reduce medication errors in the ICU by 25% within 12 months.

Examples of Effective Changes

The team at Baptist Medical Center identified several steps in the ICU's medication process that presented opportunities for error. After talking to the ICU staff about what problems they saw, the team used three change concepts—"Standardize," "Use Constraints and Forcing Functions," and "Reduce Reliance on Memory"—to develop ideas for changes in the medication process.

See Part 3, Change Concepts for Reducing Adverse Drug Events, for a complete discussion of these and other change concepts.

CHANGE 1: STANDARDIZE PHYSICIANS' ORDERS.

Change Concept
Standardize

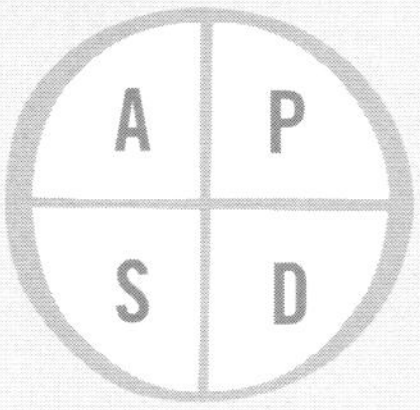

Before the change, physicians wrote orders using their own abbreviations and styles, thus creating many opportunities for error when these orders were interpreted by pharmacy staff.

After the change, physicians follow simple guidelines for writing orders. The team studied various existing order-writing guidelines, adapted them to create customized order-writing guidelines for the ICU, and disseminated the guidelines to all staff writing orders in the ICU.

The following guidelines were posted on the front of each patient's chart in the ICU:

BAPTIST MEDICAL CENTER, COLUMBIA

Guidelines for Physicians' Orders

Recommendation	Preferred	Prone to Error
Use ball point rather than felt tip pens.		
Write date and time at top of each order set.		
Write out "units"; do not abbreviate "u."	heparin 5000 units	heparin 5000 u
Do not place a decimal followed by a zero to the right of a whole number.	Ativan 1 mg	Ativan 1.0 mg
Always place a zero followed by a decimal to the left of a fraction.	digoxin 0.125 mg	digoxin .125 mg
Order medications by "mcg," "mg" or "g" strength where applicable.	Tylenol 650 mg Fer-In-Sol 125 mg	Tylenol 2 tabs Fer-In-Sol 1 cc
Avoid the use of drug name abbreviations.	penicillin sliding-scale insulin	PCN SSI
Avoid the use of QD, QID, QOD.	Q day, daily, four times daily, every other day (BID< TID q6h, q24h acceptable)	QD QID QOD
Sign your full name legibly.		

Process Measure

After the change, the pharmacy reviewed all physicians' orders from the ICU for compliance with the guidelines. Nonconforming orders dropped from an average of 15% before the process change to 9% after the change.

Baptist Medical Center, Columbia (Continued)

Examples of Effective Changes

CHANGE 2: IMPROVE MEDICATION DISPENSING AND ADMINISTRATION.

Change Concept

Use Constraints and Forcing Functions

The team made three key process changes that together altered the roles of the pharmacy and the ICU in the preparation of IV medications. All three changes introduced constraints designed to prevent errors involving high-hazard substances.

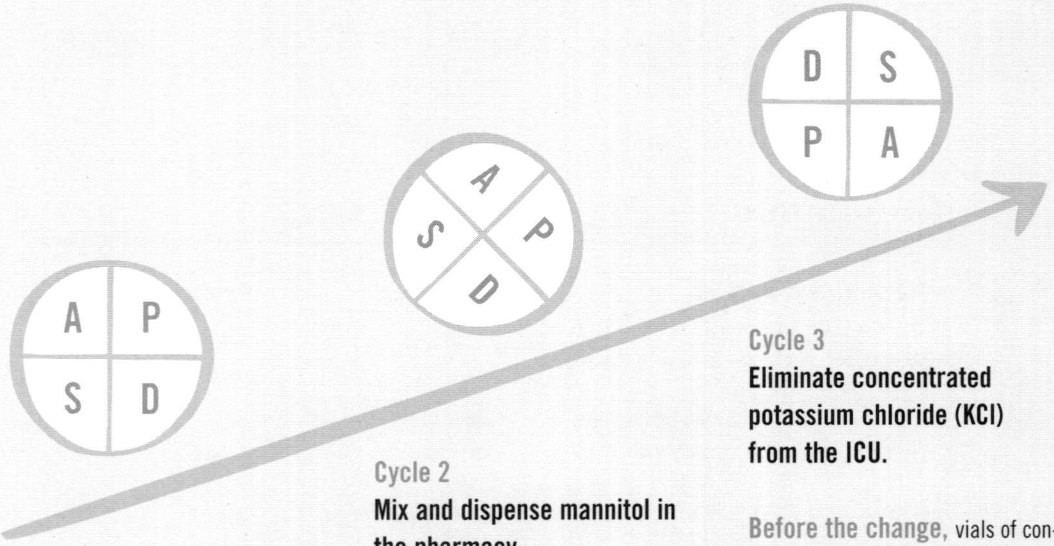

Cycle 1

Change dispensing of Solu-Medrol from IV piggyback to IV push.

Before the change, all Solu-Medrol doses greater than 20 mg were dispensed from the pharmacy as IV piggyback infusions. Nurses who preferred to administer Solu-Medrol IV push consequently had to choose between giving the piggyback and risking the excess fluid volume or mixing their own push and thus risk making a wrong-dose error.

After the change, all doses of Solu-Medrol are dispensed to the ICU as IV push. The premixed push solution is a constraint that prevents wrong-dose errors in the ICU.

Cycle 2

Mix and dispense mannitol in the pharmacy.

Before the change, the ICU obtained large-volume mannitol solutions from central supply. The ICU nurse then infused the patient with the ordered volume via IV pump and discarded the remaining volume.

After the change, the pharmacy receives the order for mannitol. The pharmacy dispenses to the ICU the exact volume ordered, labeled with the patient's name and amount. The ICU then infuses the entire volume of mannitol via IV pump. The new process creates a constraint that prevents overdose errors on the unit.

Cycle 3

Eliminate concentrated potassium chloride (KCl) from the ICU.

Before the change, vials of concentrated KCl on the unit posed a risk of lethal dose errors. In fact, one of the most common causes of fatal drug errors is accidental injection of KCl.

After the change, concentrated KCl was removed from the unit. The pharmacy dispenses all KCl to the unit, premixed in IV solutions. Requiring all IV admixture of KCl in the pharmacy introduces a constraint that reduces the risk of lethal dose errors.

CHANGE 3: MAKE INFORMATION AVAILABLE ON BRAND AND GENERIC NAMES.

Change Concept
Reduce Reliance on Memory

Relying on memory to transpose from brand to generic names of drugs created an opportunity for error.

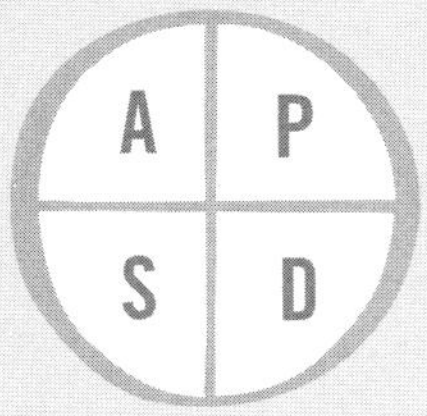

Before the change, the nursing staff would frequently go to the automated point-of-care drug-dispensing machine to obtain a drug that had been ordered by brand name but was stocked in the drug-dispensing machine by its generic name. Nurses had to remember the correct generic name to avoid a wrong-drug error.

After the change, the team created an easy-to-read alphabetic listing of drugs by brand name and by generic name and placed this list on the automated drug-dispensing machine. In this way, nurses can easily cross-reference brand and generic drug names, rather than rely on memory or leave the area to find the formulary and research the name.

RESULTS

Within 12 months, the team from Baptist Medical Center reduced the percentage of serious medication errors in the ICU from 1.67 per month to 1.18 per month—a reduction of 29%.

2 Lucile Salter Packard Children's Hospital at Stanford Palo Alto, CA

Aim: Eliminate cardiovascular drip errors in the neonatal intensive care unit (NICU) within 12 months.

Examples of Effective Changes

In the handoff when a neonate returns from surgery, the critical task of getting the cardiovascular IVs correct presented a high potential for error. The team discovered several problems: the use of different concentrations, incorrect or missing labels for the solutions, and inconsistent information on doses already given. The nursing staff reported frequent near-misses when a harmful error was only narrowly averted. Staff members agreed they must standardize practice and improve the transfer of information in this handoff.

CHANGE 1: IMPROVE THE PROCESS OF PREPARING CARDIAC IV DRIPS.

Change Concept
Standardize

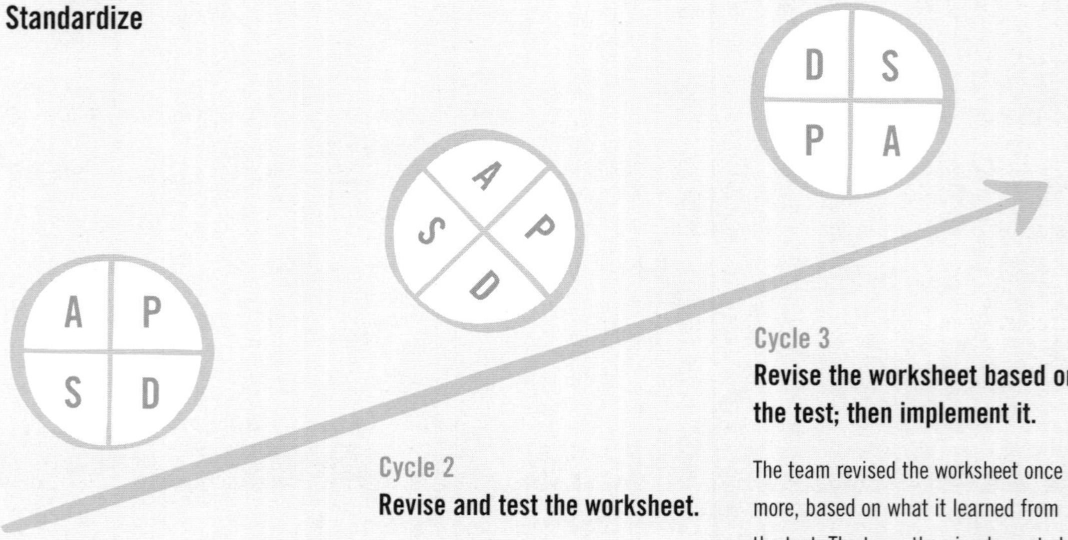

Cycle 1
Develop a standard cardiac IV drip worksheet.

The team developed a standard cardiac IV drip worksheet including concentrations, doses, and volume per kilogram for all standard cardiac medications.

Cycle 2
Revise and test the worksheet.

The cardiovascular surgery staff and anesthesia staff revised the worksheet, adding standardizations such as syringe volume and weight range cut-offs. The team then tested the worksheet on five patients.

Cycle 3
Revise the worksheet based on the test; then implement it.

The team revised the worksheet once more, based on what it learned from the test. The team then implemented the worksheet as a protocol for the administration of cardiovascular drips in all cardiovascular surgery patients.

CHANGE 2: ELIMINATE ERRORS DUE TO UNNECESSARY HANDOFFS.

Change Concepts

Reduce Handoffs

Improve Access to Information

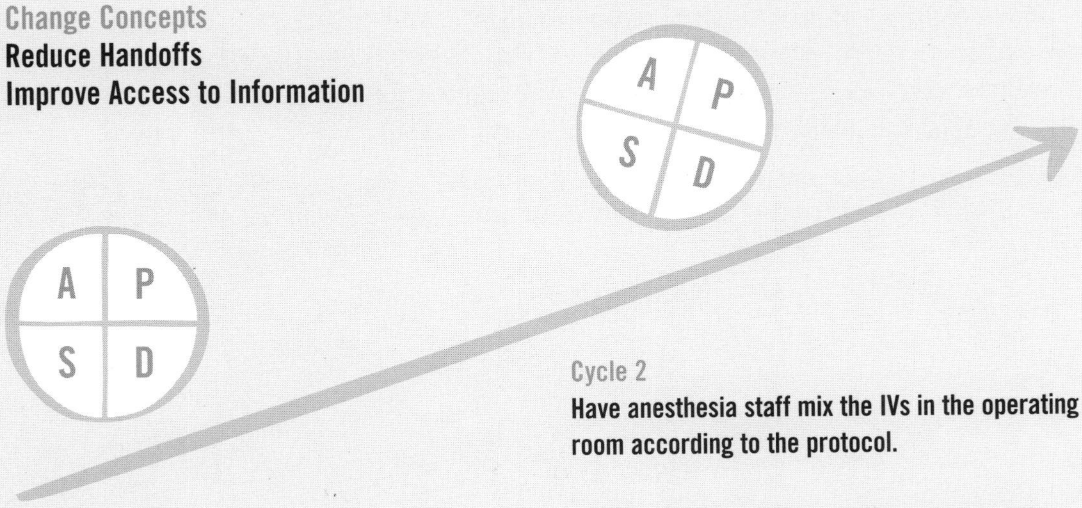

Cycle 1

Have the pharmacy produce labels for IVs preoperatively based on physician orders and according to the protocol.

Before the change, the pharmacy mixed and labeled the correct medication postoperatively, and sent it to the unit. Often the solutions were not according to protocol and had unclear labels.

After the change, the pharmacy generates the labels preoperatively, according to the protocol, and sends them to the operating room with the patient.

Cycle 2

Have anesthesia staff mix the IVs in the operating room according to the protocol.

Before the change, the nurses hung the correct IVs on the unit when the patient returned.

After the change, the anesthesia staff hangs the IVs in the operating room according to the protocol and using the labels sent up from the pharmacy. This makes it unnecessary to hang new bags on the unit and ensures that the labels are already correct.

RESULTS

Once the protocol was instituted, the fluid volume per kilogram was within the recommended range 100% of the time; labels were correct nearly 100% of the time; and the IV solutions did not need changing for 48 hours postoperatively, thus eliminating another handoff and reducing costs. Standardizing the process also improved communication between the operating room and NICU staffs, enabling them to undertake other improvements in postoperative care.

3 Pontiac Osteopathic Hospital Medical Center Pontiac, MI

Aim: Reduce adverse drug events in the cardiac monitoring unit (CMU) by 50% within 12 months.

Examples of Effective Changes

The team chose to focus on the cardiac monitoring unit because of a history of serious errors on the unit and the higher risk among these patients, who had more complex medication profiles and used more high-hazard medications. The changes selected covered different medications and procedures but fell under five change concepts: Standardize, Improve Access to Information, Optimize the Work Environment for Safety, Automate Carefully, and Simplify.

Change Concept
Standardize

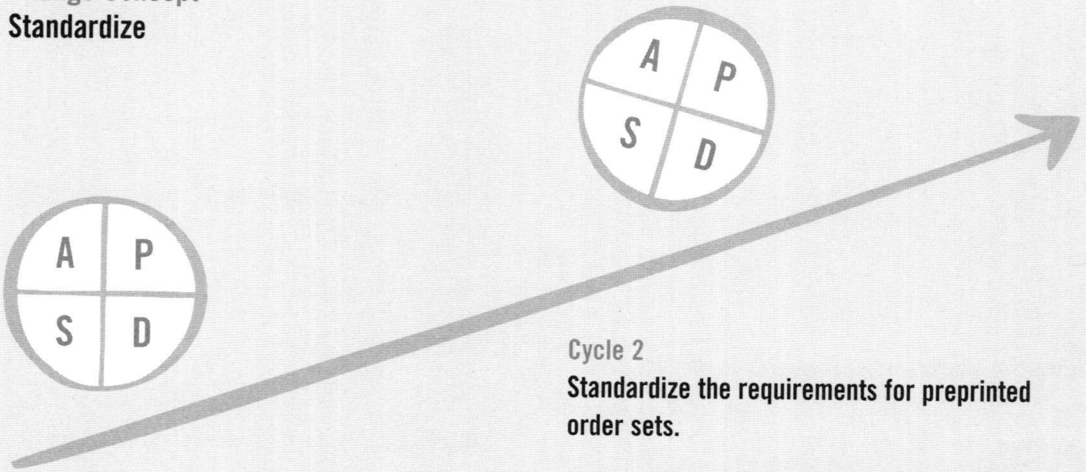

Cycle 1
Develop preprinted order sets for cardiac care in chest pain, for pneumonia, and for thrombolysis.

Several conditions were common enough to allow for standardized treatment regimens. Physicians helped develop preprinted orders for their patients with such common conditions, thus eliminating the need to continuously write the same orders. In addition, as nurses became familiar with the orders, they needed to make fewer telephone calls to clarify or change orders.

Cycle 2
Standardize the requirements for preprinted order sets.

It was clear that some order sets were easier to use than others. The team standardized the information needed for each order set and worked with physicians to modify order sets that needed improvement. In addition, the team developed preprinted orders for congestive heart failure and heparin therapy.

CHANGES

Change Concept

Improve Access to Information

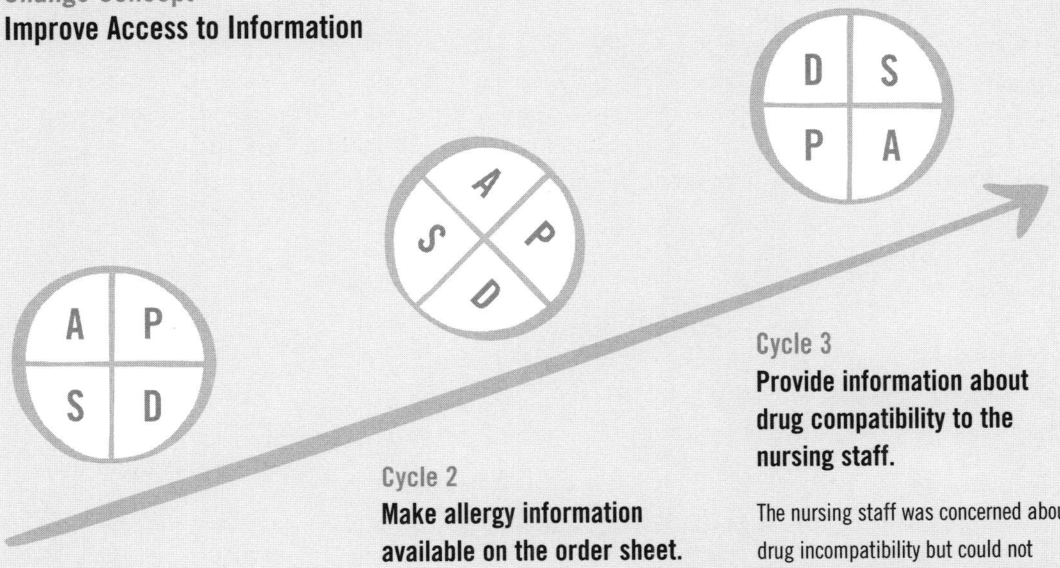

Cycle 1

Use color-coded wristbands.

The nursing staff places a red identification band on the wrists of patients with drug allergies at the time of initial assessment in the CMU, so that nurses administering medications are instantly alerted to the allergy.

Cycle 2

Make allergy information available on the order sheet.

The team decided to locate allergy information on the order sheet itself. At the time of the initial CMU assessment, the nurse sends allergy information to the hospital information system by computer. This information is inscribed on the patient's stamp plate, which is then stamped on each order sheet.

Cycle 3

Provide information about drug compatibility to the nursing staff.

The nursing staff was concerned about drug incompatibility but could not easily access the information it needed. The team placed charts of information about IV compatibility in the medication room where the IVs are set up, thus providing the staff with easy access to needed information.

Process Measure

After the changes (Cycles 1–3), accurate allergy information was available on the order sheet and on the wristband for 75% of orders.

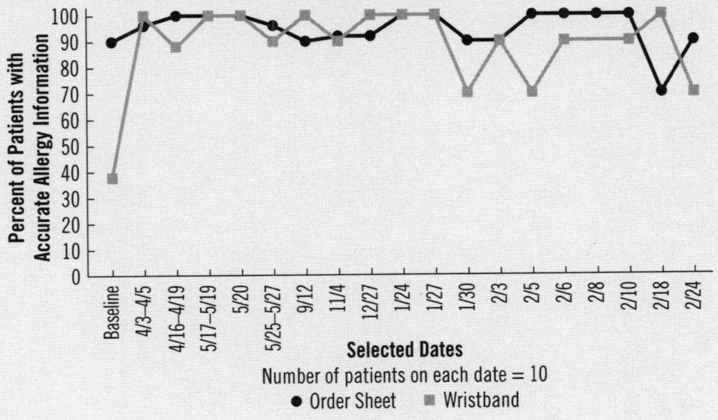

Figure 2.5

Increase in Availability of Accurate Allergy Information

Pontiac Osteopathic Hospital Medical Center (Continued)

Examples of Effective Changes

Before the changes, missing doses of IVs and other medications from the unit dose drawers presented problems for the staff. Missing doses increased the risk of omitting a medication, and at the least, wasted valuable time as staff hunted for or called for the missing medication. Discussions with the staff members indicated that these distractions interfered with their ability to feed proper information to the pharmacy technicians who fill the unit dose charts.

Change Concepts

Optimize the Work Environment for Safety
Automate Carefully

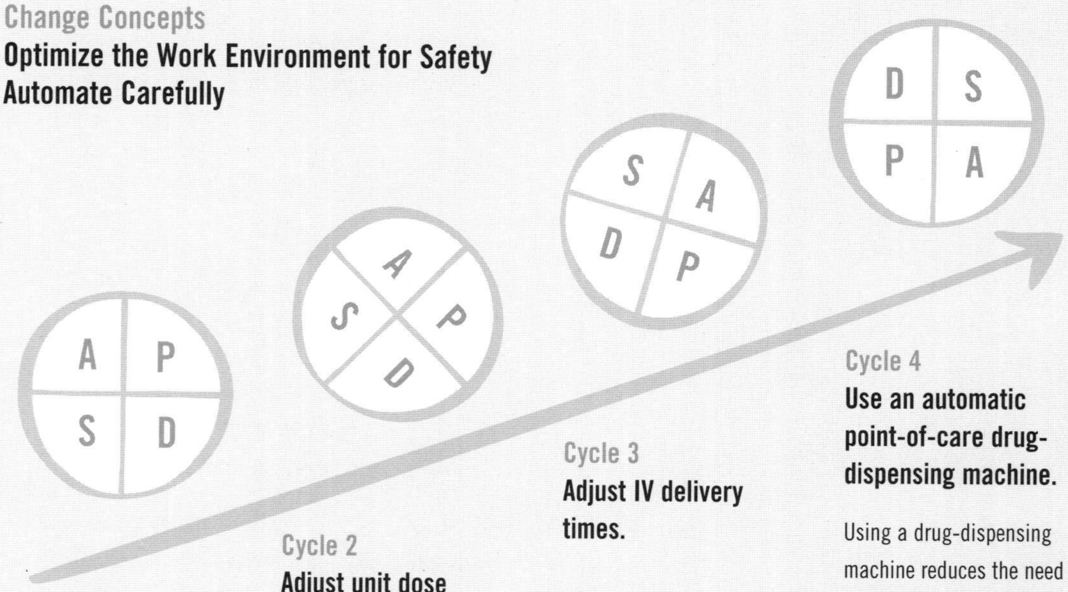

Cycle 1

Change the timing of reconciliation.

After the change, nurses reconcile the medication administration record—a critical step in filling the carts correctly—at midnight, when there are fewer distractions.

Cycle 2

Adjust unit dose delivery times.

After the change, the team adjusted the time at which the unit dose cart is changed as well as the schedule, in order to give the pharmacy technician adequate time to fill the carts carefully.

Cycle 3

Adjust IV delivery times.

After the change, IV delivery times were changed so that IV piggyback medications are readily available on the unit and on time.

Cycle 4

Use an automatic point-of-care drug-dispensing machine.

Using a drug-dispensing machine reduces the need for filling the unit dose cart, thus decreasing the chance of omissions.

Process Measure

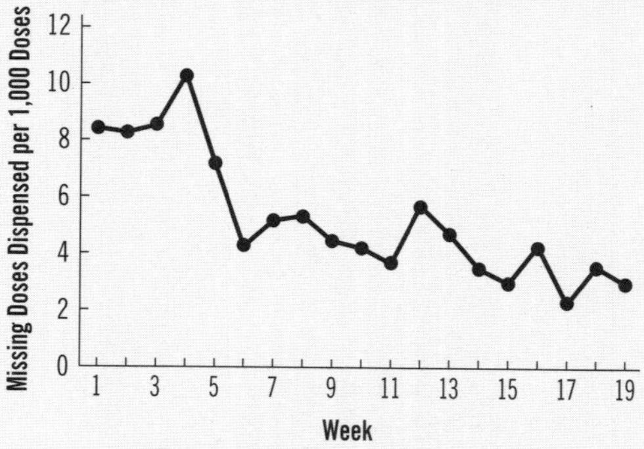

Average number of doses per week = 11,262

Figure 2.6
Reduction in Missing Doses

After the changes (Cycles 1–4), the mean number of missing doses that had to be dispensed separately from the unit dose carts decreased from 8 per 1,000 to 4 per 1,000 doses.

Change Concept

Simplify

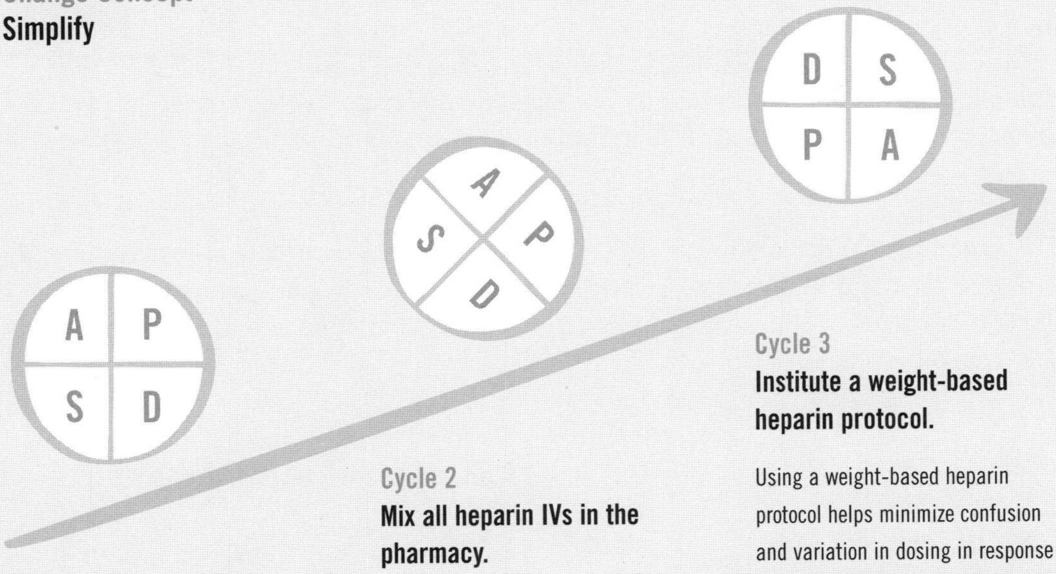

Cycle 1

To avoid dose errors, place only one concentration of heparin on the unit.

Having multiple vials of heparin available in different concentrations posed the risk of wrong-dose errors. The team decided that having only one concentration of heparin on the unit would decrease the opportunity for either an overdose or an underdose.

Cycle 2

Mix all heparin IVs in the pharmacy.

The team felt that Cycle 1 would not completely eliminate dose errors, so it decided to locate all IV admixture for heparin in the pharmacy, where there was less opportunity for error. As a result, no heparin IVs are mixed on the unit.

Cycle 3

Institute a weight-based heparin protocol.

Using a weight-based heparin protocol helps minimize confusion and variation in dosing in response to laboratory results. Physicians now use the protocol to order standard doses in response to specific laboratory results.

RESULTS

Pontiac Osteopathic Hospital's many changes led to improvement in several processes. As a result, an already declining error rate decreased further and stabilized at two serious errors per month in the Cardiac Monitoring Unit—a decrease of 80% (see Figure 2.3).

4 Promina Gwinnett Health System Lawrenceville, GA

Aim: Reduce errors in the medication ordering and administration processes by 20% within 12 months. **Intermediate Aim:** Improve the ordering and administration of heparin.

Examples of Effective Changes

This team was concerned about ordering errors in general, especially nonstandard and illegible orders, and the ordering and administration of heparin in particular. The team used several change concepts to improve the ordering and administration of heparin.

Change Concept
Reduce Handoffs

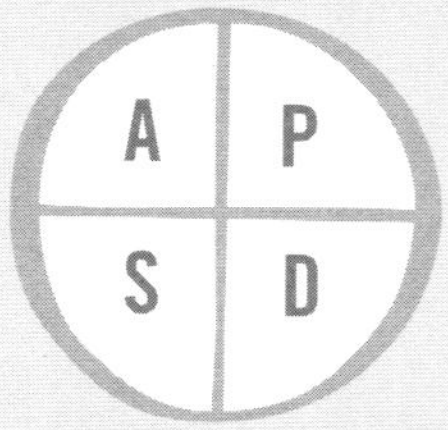

Cycle 1
Stock heparin IV and heparin bolus on unit.

Cycle time was decreased when the correct dose was already available on the unit.

Change Concept
Reduce Reliance on Memory

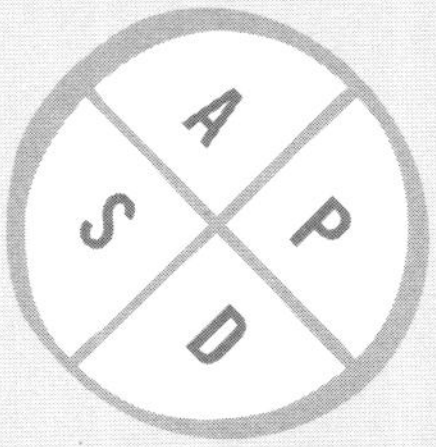

Cycle 2
Use timers to remind nurses when a heparin hold is scheduled to end.

Before the change, if the prothrombin time (aPtt) was too high, heparin was placed on hold, and the nurse had to remember to start it again in one hour. After the change, pocket timers remind nurses to restart the heparin infusion in exactly one hour.

Process Measure

Figure 2.7
Reduction in Time Between Placing the Order and Hanging the IV Bag

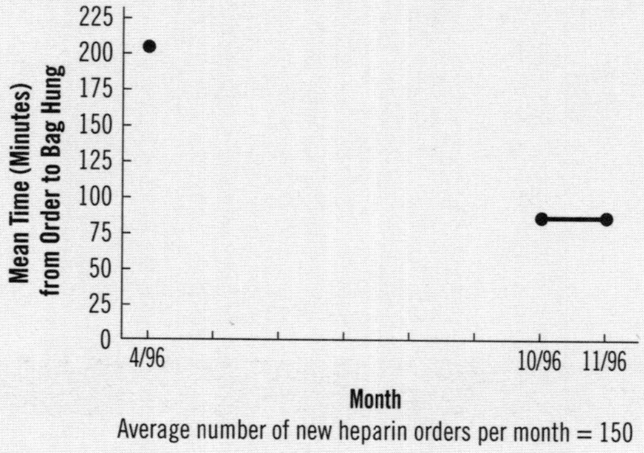

After the change (Cycle 1), the time elapsed between placing the order and hanging an IV bag with the correct dose decreased from 202 to 90 minutes.

Change Concept
Standardize

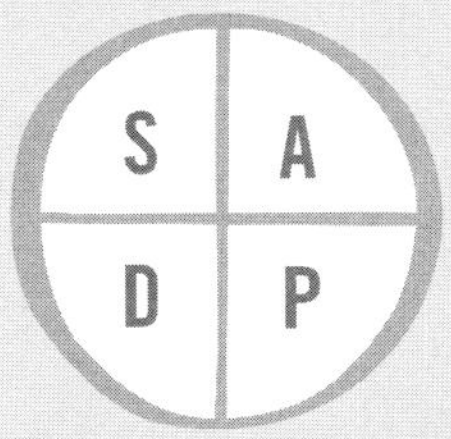

Cycle 3
Publicize a standard for performance and involve staff in finding a way to meet that standard.

The team decided to establish a minimum standard time for changing dose after receiving laboratory results. After reviewing the literature and analyzing the process, the staff set a standard of 15 minutes from results to dose change.

Change Concepts
Standardize, Simplify

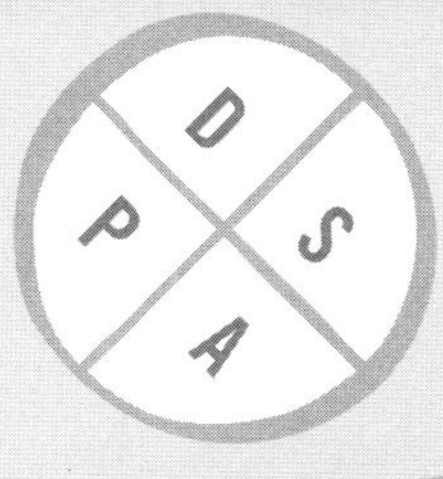

Cycle 4
Institute a weight-based heparin protocol.

Using a standard approach to initiating and maintaining anticoagulation aided the staff in adjusting the dose to aPTT levels without having to phone the physician repeatedly. Instead of having to learn several different approaches to heparin therapy, the nurses became familiar with the single approach defined in the protocol.

Process Measure

After the change (Cycle 3), the mean time elapsed between receiving laboratory results and changing the dose dropped from 29 minutes to 14 minutes.

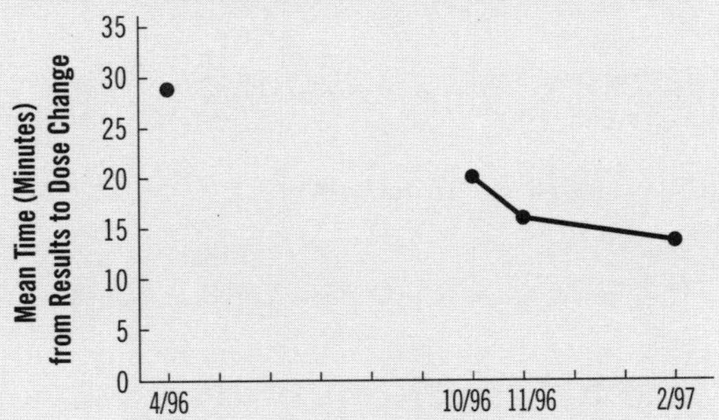

Figure 2.8
Reduction in Time Between Receiving Laboratory Results and Changing the Dose

RESULTS

The mean time to reach therapeutic aPTT for anticoagulation dropped from 24.3 hours to 14.6 hours (see Figure 2.4). The percentage of patients reaching the threshold within 24 hours increased to 100%.

Six Methods for Measuring Errors in

To improve a system, organizations must have a reliable measure of how well the system is functioning. Without reliable measures, it is impossible to tell the extent of the problem or the effect of tested changes. Health care organizations traditionally have had problems measuring errors because the primary method used—spontaneous reporting—is perceived to be inaccurate and unstable. Yet accurate and stable measures are available that allow organizations to track errors over time and to quantify the effects of changes.

Measures are used for four different purposes:

1. **Discovery** To detect errors that are occurring.

2. **Frequency estimation** To measure the frequency with which specific errors occur over time (for example, hypoglycemia).

3. **Specific measurement of a test or change** To assess the effects of changes to the system.

4. **System performance** To monitor overall system-wide errors over time.

Although no single measure is sufficient in itself to monitor the variety of systems associated with adverse drug events and medical errors, using a series of measures that combine these purposes will provide an accurate estimate of system performance over time.

Health Care

1 INSPECTION POINTS

Data collected at certain inspection points within the medication system can be used for surveillance of system performance, including the incidence of errors.

Examples of key inspection points:

- To check for discrepancies, the nurses reconcile physician orders with the medication administration record.
- To check for nonstandard orders, pharmacists process orders in the pharmacy.
- To check for missing or wrong doses, or wrong medications, the nurses administer medications using a unit dose system.

Advantages

Organizations can place stable measurement systems at specified points in the system and provide routine monitoring by key personnel such as pharmacists. Many inspection points are also "critical control points" in the medication system—points where activities occur that ensure the smooth and safe functioning of the system.

Disadvantages

- Very few.
- Inspection points do require additional time from personnel who collect the data.

Keys to optimal utilization

- Establish routine monitoring at inspection points.
- Train those involved in the inspection point on what to monitor and how to collect data.
- Review the monitoring process regularly to ensure that data is being collected appropriately.

2 FOCUS GROUPS

Focus groups are meetings to solicit ideas from those involved in a process about problems and ways to improve the process.

Advantages

Focus groups allow for direct input from those on the front line of the drug administration system: nurses, pharmacists, and physicians. These individuals have many observations and insights that are not recorded on incident reports or other methods of spontaneous reporting. Focus groups can prove an extremely useful tool for identifying system problems and "errors waiting to happen."

Disadvantages

Focus groups provide limited quantitative information on the rate of errors. Although of great value, their utility in measurement is limited to the discovery of problems.

Keys to optimal utilization

- Include those most knowledgeable about the process. To encourage a variety of perspectives, be sure that the group is diverse.
- Establish a nonpunitive environment so that participants feel free to share fully their experiences and insights.
- Choose a leader with experience in group facilitation.
- Respect opinions and observations. Take visible action following these sessions, action that demonstrates to participants that their input is helping to improve the system.

3 MONITORING OF ERROR MARKERS

Monitoring of utilization of specific items that serve as markers for errors can prevent error. An example is the use of certain antidote medications or laboratory test values that suggest when an error has occurred.

Advantages

These targeted measures can address specific problems an institution may have, such as the use of narcotics or anticoagulants. They can be monitored in a specific area (for example, in the pharmacy for antidote use or in the laboratory for specific laboratory tests or results) and on a continuous basis if desired.

Disadvantages

There are few disadvantages, if measurement is followed up to assure that an ADE did, in fact, occur.

Keys to optimal utilization

- Do not attempt to monitor all markers at all times; instead, target specific problem areas.
- Partner with the laboratory to collect and report monitored laboratory results or establish computer access to routine laboratory data and screen it regularly.
- Consider the use of these drugs or the presence of certain lab values as possible indicators of error, and investigate to ascertain if a real error did occur.

Markers of Possible ADEs and Errors

Drug use that might be markers of an adverse drug event:

- activated charcoal
- Digibind
- diphenhydramine
- diphenoxylate/atropine
- hydroxyzine
- Kayexalate
- naloxone
- protamine
- Romazicon
- steroid cream
- vitamin K
- loperamide

Laboratory results that might be markers of error:

- digoxin levels
- glucose levels (plasma) less than about 50 (exact level to be determined by individual organizations)
- potassium levels (plasma) greater than about five (exact level to be determined by individual organizations)
- PT/PTT/INRs
- theophylline levels

4 CHART REVIEW

A focused, in-depth review of medical records can identify medical errors. Chart review includes all available information contained within the medical record (physician and nursing notes, orders, laboratory results, and radiology reports) and is usually augmented with interviews of staff regarding questionable events.

Advantages

Trained observers can spot errors that are not identified by spontaneous reporting.

Disadvantages

- There is a danger of overlooking data: Evidence of error might be subtle, requiring that one read between the lines. An abnormal lab result may be the only clue.
- Thorough review takes time.
- Variation exists among chart reviewers.

Keys to optimal utilization

- Use knowledgeable chart review personnel and case investigators—generally nurses or pharmacists.
- Train chart review personnel and case investigators adequately.

5 OBSERVATION

A trained observer can watch a process as it takes place in order to detect errors.

Advantages

- Observation has the highest yield of any detection method (2 to 3 times greater yield than chart review, 20 to 30 times greater yield than spontaneous reporting).
- Observers identify the steps in the process where errors occur.

Disadvantages

- The presence of an observer may alter the behavior of those being observed. This is a transient effect, of little significance, provided that the observer does not give advice or participate in any way.
- Because of variable observation skills, different observers may capture different information.
- Observer inference may occur, leading to misinterpretation of what is seen; this is a function of observer bias, knowledge, and experience and can be minimized by training.
- Careful specification is needed in order to achieve uniform recording of data.

Keys to optimal utilization

- Use observers who are experienced and sophisticated enough (generally nurses or pharmacists) to understand what is being done and recognize when there is a variance.
- Train observers thoroughly and provide them with in-depth knowledge of the processes being observed.
- Choose the right process to observe.

6 SPONTANEOUS REPORTING

Routine use of incident or error report forms completed by health care personnel to report adverse events can quickly reduce errors. A simple form like the one on the facing page fits onto a 5 in. × 7 in. card. Blank cards (shown opposite in reduced size) can be kept in clinical areas for easy access. The reporting person fills out Side 1. The investigating person fills out Side 2.

Advantages

Most health care organizations already use incident or error reporting.

Disadvantages

- Reporting is inconsistent, and even in the best of circumstances organizations have a difficult time assuring consistency.
- Reporting is ambiguous.
- Reporting typically yields limited data; the method has punitive overtones and generally requires additional work from busy staff members.

Keys to optimal utilization

- Create a nonpunitive reporting environment.
- Use reporting for improvement rather than for judgment.
- Make reporting anonymous.
- Reward reporting.
- Use a simple report form, which requires minimal time and effort to complete.
- Clearly define what should be reported.
- Customize reporting criteria and report forms for specific locations such as general medical wards, pharmacy, and intensive care units.
- Provide clear evidence of follow-up from reports, including process changes implemented as a result.
- Plan for the limitations of spontaneous reporting. Supplement it with other types of data.

Sample Spontaneous Reporting Form

◄ **Side 1** is filled out by the individual **reporting** the event.

Adverse Drug Reactions and Adverse Drug Events Reporting Form

Patient Name ______________________________

Medical Record Number ______________ Date of Report ______________

Reporting Individual: 1. ☐ nurse 2. ☐ pharmacist 3. ☐ physician
4. ☐ other ______________________________

Classification of the event (check one):

1. ☐ ADR (adverse drug reaction): An unexpected reaction (not a side effect) to a drug that was used in a proper manner. No error was involved (includes non-preventable ADEs).
2. ☐ Preventable ADE (adverse drug event): An injury due to an error in the use of a drug (including failure to use).
3. ☐ Medication error with no potential for injury.
4. ☐ Potential ADE (adverse drug event): A medication error with the potential to cause injury.

The event occurred on: Date ________ Time ______________ (am/pm) Nursing Unit

Name of medication: ______________________________

Route administered: 1. ☐ PO 2. ☐ IV 3. ☐ IM 4. ☐ other __________

Brief description of event: ______________________________

____

____

◄ **Side 2** is filled out by the individual **investigating** the event.

Investigating Instructions:
Complete the following information for all errors.

Stage in the medication process where the error occurred (check one):

1. ☐ Ordering
2. ☐ Transcription
3. ☐ Dispensing
4. ☐ Administration
5. ☐ Documentation

Type of error(s) involved (check all that apply):

A. ☐ Wrong dose
B. ☐ Wrong route
C. ☐ Wrong frequency (or rate for IV)
D. ☐ Wrong drug
E. ☐ Wrong choice
F. ☐ Wrong time
G. ☐ Wrong administration technique
H. ☐ Missed dose
I. ☐ Known drug-drug interaction
J. ☐ Known allergy to drug
K. ☐ Other

THUS FAR IN THE GUIDE, YOU HAVE LEARNED:

Part 1 *The Model for Improvement, which can be applied to any area you want to improve.*

Part 2 *A step-by-step guide to using the model to work on reducing adverse drug events, with each of the basic steps—setting aims, forming the team, establishing measures, and developing and testing changes—illustrated with examples.*

Part 3

Change Concepts for Reducing Adverse Drug Events

In this section, you will learn a group of change concepts that can be applied in different ways throughout the medication system—in the ordering, dispensing, and administration processes—to reduce adverse drug events.

Part 3 is conceptual:

- It provides a framework for understanding different **causes of errors** in health care.
- It introduces **change concepts for preventing errors** in health care.

Part 4 is practical:

- It explains **how to apply the change concepts** to improve the medication system.

Preventing Errors in Health Care

Even highly trained people make mistakes.

Error prevention in health care has relied almost exclusively on the training of personnel to perform perfectly, reinforced by punishment when personnel performance fails. The operative concept is that highly trained people do not make errors. Unfortunately, this is not true.

Cognitive psychologists and human factors specialists have long recognized that human beings are incapable of consistent error-free performance (see Reason, *Human Error*, 1990, and Perrow, *Normal Accidents*, 1984). More importantly, they have shown that the systems in which people work have a marked effect on the incidence of human error. For example, "look-alike" labels and "sound-alike" names are medication accidents waiting to happen. Although conscientious and highly trained people, such as nurses, pharmacists, and physicians, take pains to be careful, sooner or later they will make a mistake and a patient will receive the wrong drug.

Preventing errors requires designing systems better.

Effective prevention of errors, therefore, requires designing systems to incorporate human factors principles. *Human factors principles* are concepts about the design of work that take advantage of the strengths of the human mind and compensate for its limitations. They include practices such as standardization, simplification, and reducing reliance on memory. This Guide refers to such principles as change concepts. Applying these principles to the design of work reduces the likelihood of error.

Industrial Models

A number of industries outside of health care have developed and implemented the concept of preventing errors by correcting and preventing system failures. The most notable example is the aviation industry. Airlines strive for "zero defects." Like physicians, pilots are highly trained and held to high standards of performance. But in contrast to medicine, airlines, aircraft manufacturers, and the Federal Aviation Authority (FAA) have learned that relying solely on training and standards will not prevent accidents. To ensure safety, the airline industry, using human factors principles, has developed a wide array of systemic and organizational safeguards.

For example:

Standardization is widely employed for procedures, equipment, and tasks.

Fail-safe mechanisms correct for possible failures of equipment or errors in performance.

Forcing functions make many errors impossible.

Instruments and organized support systems supply accurate and extensive information.

Monitoring is extensive and, should an instrument fail, available in duplicate or triplicate.

Automation, used wherever possible, further reduces the risk of human error.

Teamwork is encouraged among pilots and other members of the crew.

Strict regulations ensure that crews are not overworked or fatigued.

The results achieved by the airlines are impressive. For passengers, the risk of a fatal crash is one in 2 million. Airlines are truly "high-reliability" organizations. Health care can learn a great deal from aviation.

Causes of Errors in Health Care

Health care is complex, involving the interaction of large numbers of highly trained personnel in many diverse, interrelated, and interdependent activities. This Guide refers to these activities as systems. System failures can be grouped into two broad categories: design failures and organizational failures.

DESIGN FAILURES

Most errors made by individuals at the "sharp end" (i.e., where the action occurs) result from failures in the design of systems and components (see Reason, 1990). These system failures usually occur in a time and space far removed from the actual error. Many hospital systems inadvertently induce errors because they were never "designed" in the true sense, but just grew and developed without reference to human factors principles. Design failures fall into three categories: failures of process design, task design, and equipment design.

Process design failures

Faulty processes induce errors and make errors difficult to detect in time to prevent injury. Many design failures result from a failure to think through the purposes of the process and how best to achieve those purposes.

Planners neglect to ask basic questions:

- What are the objectives of the process?
- How can the process best meet users' needs?
- What are the potential hazards of this process?
- What are the "What if?"s—the consequences of actions that can go wrong?

ORGANIZATIONAL FAILURES

In contrast to design failures, which relate to specifics of how individuals perform complex tasks, organizational failures affect the broader psychological and sociological aspects of how individuals function. Clearly, the two are interrelated, and organizational factors are also "designed." However, unlike design failures, organizational failures can sometimes be remedied by "low-level" changes that can be implemented in a relatively short time, often as pilot projects, without the need for substantial additional resources. Careful consideration of three types of organizational factors—psychological precursors, team functioning, and training—can help reduce adverse drug events.

Psychological precursors

Psychological precursors are workplace conditions. As James Reason has pointed out in his classic work, *Human Error* (New York: Cambridge University Press; 1990), schedules, work assignments, relationships, and environmental factors can cause sleep loss, fatigue, and other forms of stress that increase the likelihood of errors. Examples of potentially harmful workplace conditions include unreasonable work schedules that require too much time or contain too many tasks, poor environmental conditions (inadequate heat, light, space), and fear in the workplace.

Task design failures

Many common tasks are not "user-friendly"—that is, they rely on cognitive functions that are known to be weak and error-prone (for example, short-term memory), and they don't incorporate design features that have been shown to reduce errors. As a result, they permit or even induce errors. Basic human factors principles such as standardization, simplification, and forcing functions have not been used as well and as widely as they could be.

Equipment design failures

This is the "hard-core" human factors area: the human-machine interface. While health care systems frequently require the use of complicated equipment (for example, anesthesia machines, ventilators, IV pumps), users are seldom provided with easy-to-understand information and controls. Designers of hospital equipment have, in many cases, failed to apply basic human factors principles. It is not an exaggeration to say that, with the possible exception of anesthesiologists, most of the personnel using most hospital equipment do not understand how to use it, in the sense of understanding its functions, how to adjust the equipment, and what error signals mean. In large part, operator failures result from unnecessarily complex displays and controls and the absence of forcing functions (for example, attachments that make it impossible to attach enteral tubes to IV connectors).

Team functioning

Interactions among personnel have a significant impact on individual performance. A supportive environment combined with skilled leadership will encourage individuals to work well with one another, help each other avoid mistakes, intercept errors, and improve the work environment. To be effective, teams must develop communication and leadership skills, group norms, and a sense of group cohesion. Teams are likely to be less effective where doctors and nurses have traditionally functioned in a semiautonomous manner, or where managers frequently use autocratic methods and blame as management tools.

Training

Typically, the only response to error is increased training for the person who made the error. But the response needs to be broader. Since training issues often underlie poor performance, the organization should make sure all personnel receive training needed to prevent errors. To the extent that personnel lack skills and understanding of their tasks and responsibilities, they will be more likely to make errors. Competence is the first requirement in error prevention.

Change Concepts for Reducing Adverse

See Part 4, Achieving Breakthrough Improvement in Reducing Adverse Drug Events, for examples of how organizations in the Breakthrough Series Collaborative applied these change concepts to reduce adverse drug events.

The following are change concepts that organizations can use to reduce adverse drug events. The concepts and examples introduced in this section are distilled from the scientific literature on error, both inside and outside health care. They represent the strategies that have proven most effective in reducing adverse drug events. The organizations in the Breakthrough Series Collaborative used these change concepts as a starting point for their work.

The change concepts are grouped in two general categories:

- **PROCESS DESIGN**
  Refining and redesigning what we do
- **ORGANIZATIONAL CHANGE**
  Redesigning how we do it

Drug Events

PROCESS DESIGN

1 Reduce Reliance on Memory
2 Simplify
3 Standardize
4 Use Constraints and Forcing Functions
5 Use Protocols and Checklists Wisely
6 Improve Access to Information
7 Decrease Reliance on Vigilance
8 Reduce Handoffs
9 Decrease Multiple Entry
10 Differentiate: Eliminate Look-alikes and Sound-alikes
11 Automate Carefully

ORGANIZATIONAL CHANGE

12 Optimize the Work Environment for Safety
13 Increase Feedback
14 Train for Teamwork
15 Drive Out Fear
16 Obtain Leadership Commitment
17 Improve Direct Communication

Using a Change Concept to Develop and

A change concept is a general idea—with proven merit and a sound scientific or logical foundation—that can stimulate specific ideas for changes that lead to improvement. As a theoretically grounded idea used to organize a series of small-scale Plan-Do-Study-Act (PDSA) cycles, the change concept is the driving connection between each small change an organization makes and its larger goal of breakthrough improvement.

- The **change concept** is the theoretically grounded idea for change.
- The **process change** is the specific application of that idea to a process within the medication system.
- The **Plan-Do-Study-Act (PDSA) cycle** tests the process change to see if it leads to improvement.

Test a Process Change

▶ Here's how one organization used a change concept to develop and test a process change

Aim
Reduce adverse drug events in the Intensive Care Unit.

Change Concept
Standardize

Process Change
Standardize the administration of IV potassium chloride (KCl).

Plan-Do-Study-Act (PDSA) Cycle

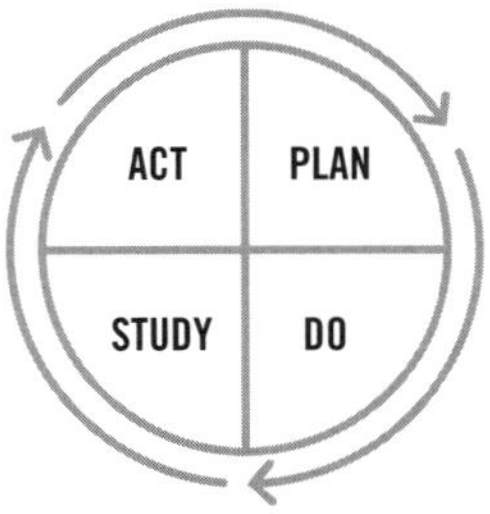

Plan

- Stock only standard, premixed IV solutions on the unit instead of concentrated KCl in vials.
- Assess the availability of concentrated KCl on the unit.
- Measure the number of times KCl administration was delayed.
- Prediction: Standardized and simplified administration of IV potassium chloride will reduce potential adverse drug events.

Do

Carry out plan and collect data.

Study

- No concentrated KCl was available on the unit.
- Because pharmacists were unfamiliar with the new process, administration was delayed in 10% of doses, requiring special delivery from the pharmacy.

Act

- Implement the change as tested.
- Work with the pharmacy on decreasing the time it takes to make solutions available and on increasing the floor stock.

Change Concepts for **Process Design**

Poorly functioning processes should sometimes be entirely discarded (see Michael Hammer, *Reengineering the Corporation: A Manifesto for Business Revolution*. New York, NY: Harper Business; 1993). Consider this option seriously if a process is functioning poorly and if the institution's leadership is willing to make the creation and design of a new process a priority. Generally, however, improving the process is the more feasible option. The objective is to redesign the process so that failures are nearly impossible or at least to incorporate features into the design that make it possible to detect an error in time to prevent patient injury.

1 Reduce Reliance on Memory

Memory, both long- and short-term, is one of the more fallible human cognitive functions. Many tasks in health care require some degree of memory (for example, a physician remembering that the patient has renal failure or a nurse remembering to give a medication at a specific time). As much as possible, design medication processes to minimize reliance on memory by, for example, including in the processes automatic prompts to guide or correct action.

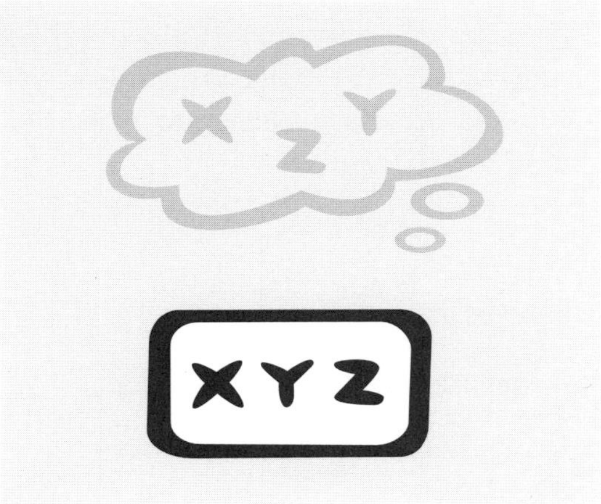

Changes that reduce reliance on memory:

- Use drug-drug interaction checking systems.
- Use computerized order entry.
- Use guided dose algorithms.
- Use laminated dosing cards to help remember tasks.
- Use bar coding on drugs (containers and doses), medication records, and patient wristbands.
- Use computerized patient information.
- Use computerized drug dispensing.
- Use timers or alarms.

Examples:

- Many pharmacies use computerized checking systems to identify drug-drug interactions.
- Several organizations print dosing algorithms on order sheets for antibiotics, chemotherapeutics, heparin, parenteral nutrition, and other medications to help physicians calculate the dose.
- Some organizations use laminated dosing cards to help with a variety of memory tasks. Cards can include standard order times, standard doses of antibiotics, formulas for calculating pediatric doses, and common chemotherapy protocols.
- One organization hung small digital timers on the doors of patients' rooms to remind nurses when to change specific IV piggyback medications.

2 Simplify

The antidote for complexity is simplification. Most processes are more complicated than they need to be. For example, the medication system in an average hospital involves 15 to 20 steps and as many as a dozen different people. Fewer steps lead to fewer errors. Every step in a complicated process provides an opportunity for error. Simplicity makes the process easier to understand and errors easier to recognize. Make processes as elemental as possible by eliminating unnecessary steps.

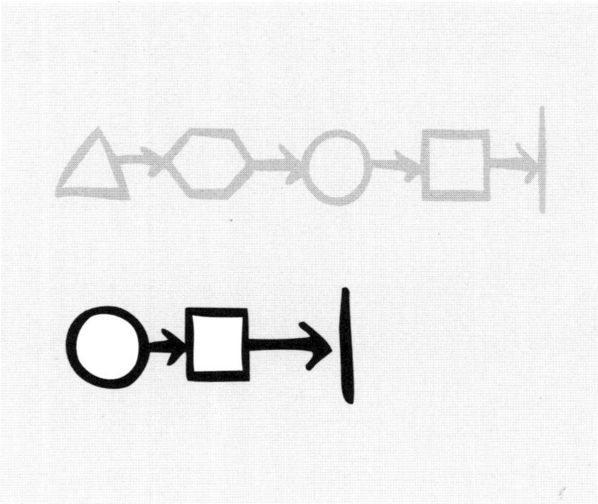

Changes that simplify:

- Eliminate transcription of orders.
- Limit choices of available drugs in the pharmacy.
- Limit the dosage strengths and concentrations for each drug (use a maximum of two).
- Maintain inventory of frequently used prepared drugs, rather than preparing such drugs to order.
- Limit the number of times per day that drugs are administered.
- Mix IVs in the pharmacy.
- Use a single record entry for medications.
- Automate dispensing on the unit.
- Seek equipment that has simple instructions and a convenient user interface.

Examples:

- Several organizations have limited the heparin solutions available on the nursing units to one concentration to avoid confusion and eliminate the chance of using a more concentrated dose by mistake.
- Many organizations have restricted the number of protocols for the same medication so that the staff can become familiar with just one, thus decreasing the likelihood of error.
- In several organizations, the pharmacy mixed batches of the most often used solutions each day, or once or twice a week, so that only a few had to be mixed to order during the press of a busy day.

3 Standardize

Standardization reduces the opportunities for error. If you do something the same way every time, you are less likely to do it wrong any time. For example, fewer dosing errors will occur with a drug that is only available in two strengths than with drugs doctors can order in several strengths. Similarly, there is no medical justification for multiple sliding scales for insulin. Standardizing doses reduces errors and promotes the on-time administration of drugs.

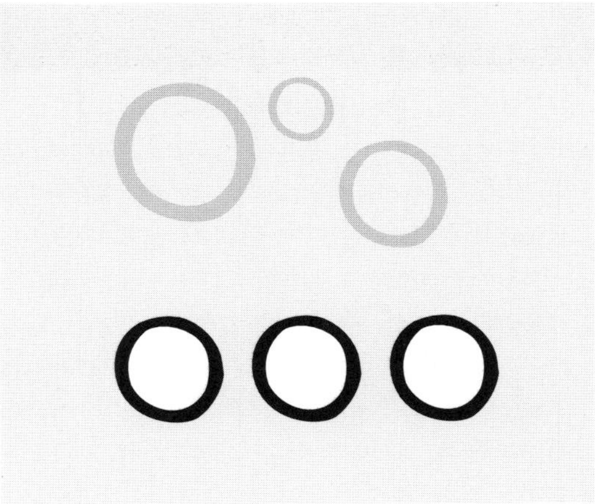

Changes that standardize:

- Standardize prescribing conventions:
  Use no abbreviations.
  Use "units" not "u".
  Use leading zero (0.5, not .5), but avoid trailing zero (5, not 5.0).
  Use generic names.
  Use metric system only.
  Do not use Q or q.
- Use protocols for complex medication administration (heparin, insulin, chemotherapy).
- Limit the number of standard doses of medication.
- Standardize times of drug administration.
- Store medications in the same place in every medication room.
- Standardize packaging and labeling for all medications (make "like" drugs look alike and differentiate drugs that are different).
- Use standard equipment, for example, one kind of pump or syringe.

Examples:

- Almost every organization established some type of protocol for medication administration.
- Many organizations set standards for prescribing practices, including appropriate abbreviations and notations.
- Several organizations standardized antibiotic administration times to prevent omissions.

4 Use Constraints and Forcing Functions

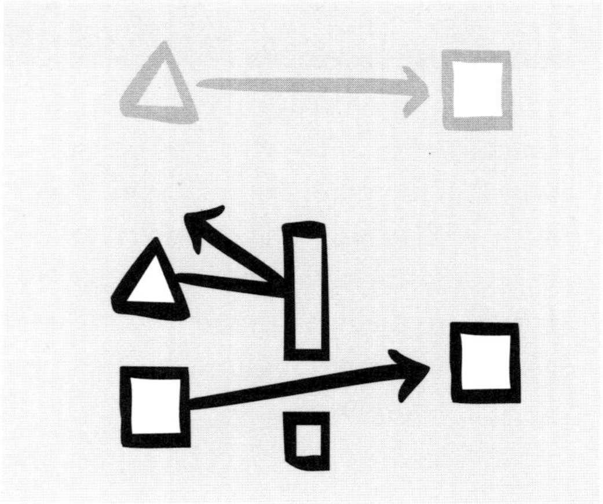

A forcing function (such as a device that makes it impossible to start a car in reverse gear) is an effective error-proofing method that eliminates relying on memory, checklists, and double check systems. Forcing functions, which can be applied to many simple tasks and are usually well accepted by personnel, make it impossible to make certain errors. For example, the design of the connections for oxygen and nitrous oxide on anesthesia machines makes it impossible to connect one to the other. Similarly, a constraint prevents further action until some condition is met (for example, a pharmacy computer that will not permit dispensing of a dose of medication unless the patient's weight is entered into the system, thus decreasing wrong-dose errors).

Changes that use constraints and forcing functions:

- Use pharmacy computers that will not fill any orders unless allergy information and patient weight and height are entered.
- Add special luer-locks to syringes and indwelling lines that have to match before fluid can be infused, thus preventing personnel from infusing non-IV solutions into IVs, central lines, or intrathecal lines.
- Use computerized order entry with range checks on doses to prevent completion of an order until the dose specified is in a safe range for the medication and the patient.
- Remove concentrated potassium chloride solutions from floor stock, thus preventing accidental rapid IV infusion of a concentrated solution or a preparation error.

Example:

- In the operating room, oxygen and nitrous oxide have separate color codes and a lock-and-key connection between the tank and the tube connecting to the patient. This makes it impossible to connect nitrous oxide to the oxygen tubing.

5 Use Protocols and Checklists Wisely

Think of protocols and checklists as memory aids rather than as rigid molds for unthinking behavior. Protocols convey information simultaneously to everyone involved about correct actions, thus decreasing the time needed for communication. They support standardization. Checklists serve as reminders of critical tasks, especially when an omission can have serious consequences. Both of these are helpful in reducing individual variation in practice, but they must be used with care, since indiscriminate adherence can also be a source of error.

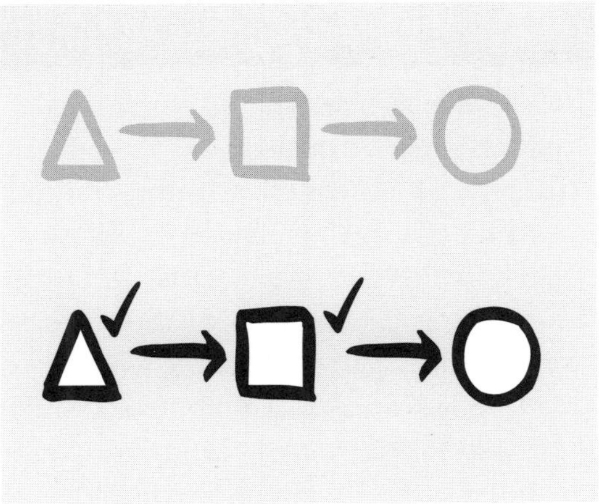

Changes for using protocols and checklists:

- Avoid statements that contain negatives (for example, "Check to see that the light is off" is better than "Check to see that the light is not on").
- Make instructions agree with the most likely state of the system—so that a "yes" is the usual response.
- Make sure that everyone has agreed on the protocol or checklist and is aware that it is in use.
- Revisit the protocol or checklist regularly to understand what exceptions were made and why. Such exceptions may require revision of the protocol or checklist.

Examples:

- Many hospitals use protocols for the administration of medications like heparin and insulin—drugs that can be lethal and have a range of doses.
- Some hospitals use checklists for high-hazard situations —preoperatively, when giving chemotherapy and administering blood products—to ensure that all information is available and all preparations have been made.
- Several organizations treat protocols as living documents. Continually evaluate and update them as needed.

6 Improve Access to Information

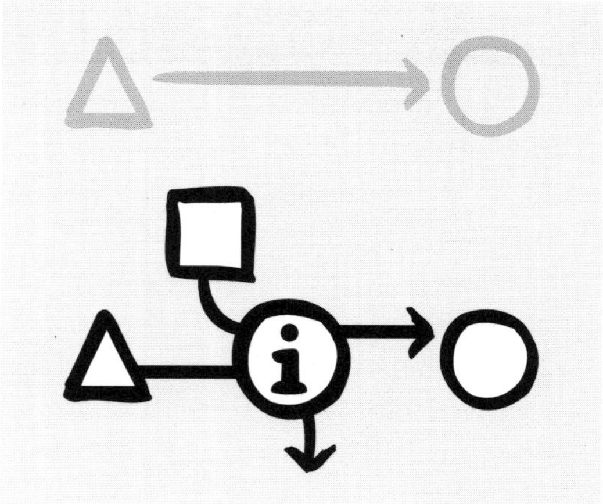

Lack of information is a common cause of errors. Many patients receive medications to which they have known allergies simply because the doctor or nurse didn't have adequate information at the time the medication was ordered or given. Doctors, nurses, pharmacists, and other personnel need to have information on medications, patients, and the results of treatment when it is needed, where it is needed, in a form that can be readily used. Computerization of patient, drug, and laboratory information holds great promise in this area, but simpler methods can also work. Likewise, organizations must make information concerning errors and system operations accessible in order to change practice and prevent errors.

Changes that improve access to information:

- Have a pharmacist available on the nursing units and at rounds.
- Use computerized order entry systems.
- Use computerized patient information.
- Use computerized laboratory data to immediately alert clinicians about abnormal lab values.
- Place lab reports and medication records at the bedside.
- Place protocols and ordering information on the patient's chart and in the medication room where they are easily accessible.
- Color-code wristbands for patients with allergies.
- Provide each patient with a list of his or her medications, doses, and times.
- Track errors or near misses and report these to staff on a weekly basis.
- Accelerate lab turnaround times for blood coagulation tests (partial thromboplastin time, or PTTs) and blood sugar tests.

Examples:

- One organization moved the medications and the medication administration record (MAR) to the bedside to make it easier to see what was needed for the patient.
- One organization began placing a red identification wristband on patients with drug allergies.
- In another organization, each patient received a list of his or her medications daily. When the nurse came to administer medications, the nurse reviewed the list with the patient.

7 Decrease Reliance on Vigilance

It is well known that there are limits to the human attention span. Fatigue, repetitive tasks, and infrequently occurring events make it particularly difficult to maintain vigilance. Anesthesiologists, for example, use specific techniques such as documenting the patient's vital signs every 5 minutes to maintain their attention to the patient's condition throughout a long surgical procedure. Change the work design to reduce requirements for focused attention that are of longer duration than most people find comfortable.

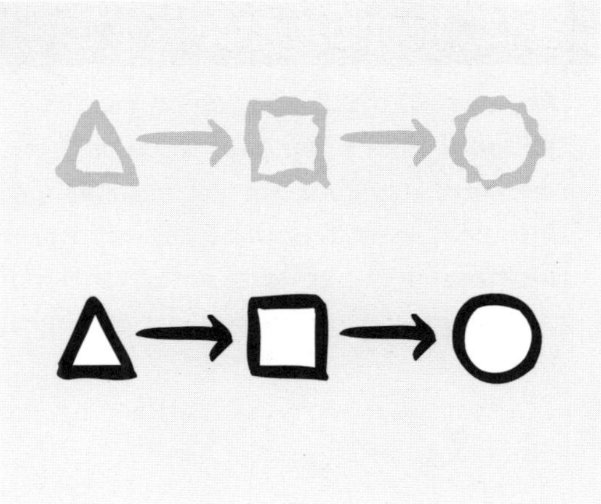

Changes that decrease reliance on vigilance:

- Use automatic drug dose checking in high-risk situations.
- Use double checks for doses of narcotics, insulin, heparin, chemotherapy, and other lethal drugs.
- Have the pharmacist monitor highly toxic drugs on a daily basis.
- Use checklists, and standardize their use at regular intervals (for example, check temperature every 15 minutes for blood products).
- Use electronic monitors that signal an alarm when parameters are exceeded, but use them carefully—they do not substitute for attention.
- Limit long shifts for physicians, nurses, and pharmacists.
- Rotate staff when performing repetitive functions.

Examples:

- Many organizations use a double check system: The nurse administering blood products or insulin shows another nurse the order and the dose and explains how it was calculated.
- Some hospitals use a clinical pharmacist to monitor daily the use of high-hazard substances on specific units.
- Some hospitals use chemotherapy double check systems for prescribers, nurses, and pharmacists.

8 Reduce Handoffs

Part of the complexity in the medication system is a result of the number of people involved and the handoffs among them. Many errors occur during the transfer of materials, information, people, instructions, or supplies. Processes that reduce the number of handoffs reduce the chances for such slips. Study a process and eliminate all unnecessary handoffs.

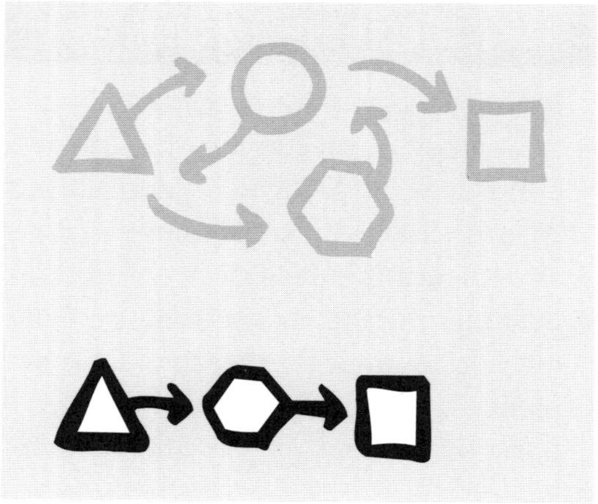

Changes that reduce handoffs:

- Provide ready-to-administer products.
- Reduce transcription of medical orders.
- Use unit dosing systems.
- Have a pharmacist participate in rounds.
- Use automated point-of-care drug delivery systems.
- Use computerized prescriber order entry.
- Use a satellite pharmacy.

Examples:

- In some organizations, point-of-care delivery systems stock up to 70% of the most commonly used medications on each nursing unit, and nurses are able to access the medications based on physicians' orders.
- Several organizations have begun to include a clinical pharmacist on the nursing units to consult with physicians about specific medications, making it easier to get the order right the first time.

9 Decrease Multiple Entry

Recording information in more than one place increases the likelihood of error.

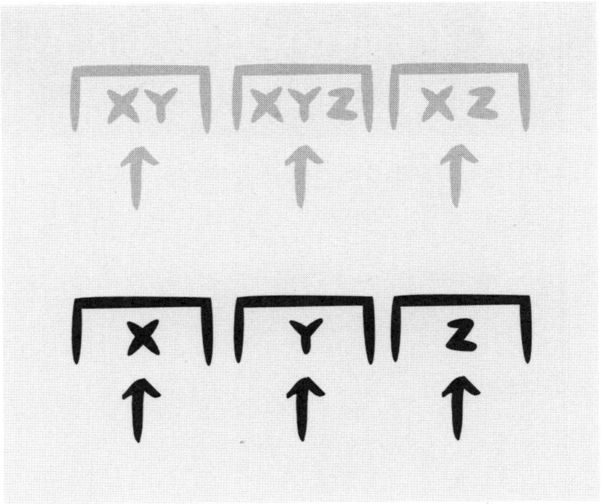

Changes that decrease multiple entry:

- Use a computerized prescriber order entry that automatically transmits the physician's order to both the pharmacy and the nursing station.
- Have the pharmacy generate a computerized medication administration record.

Example:

- One hospital implemented a computerized medication administration record system.

10 Differentiate: Eliminate Look-alikes and Sound-alikes

Similarity of packaging and labeling can cause mix-ups in the use of drugs. For example, two doses of heparin that look exactly alike except for the notation of the concentration on the label will get mixed up on some occasion. Repackage or relabel look-alike medications in a manner that highlights differences.

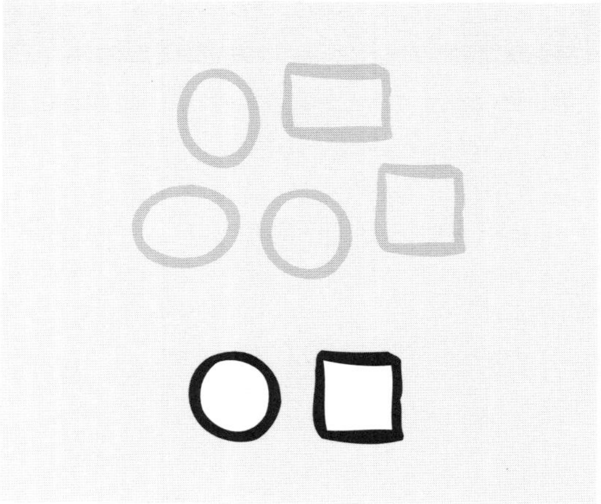

Changes that eliminate look-alikes and sound-alikes:

- Repackage or relabel look-alike medications to differentiate them.
- Store similar-looking medications in separate places.
- Alert staff and post information on sound-alike medications. (Some organizations avoid sound-alikes by using the brand name for one medication and the generic name for the other.)
- Avoid stocking look-alike packages.

Examples:

- One organization that stocked two concentrations of morphine sulfate in identical cartridges had the pharmacy label the higher-concentration cartridge with bright orange tape.
- Another organization elected to store two concentrations of IV heparin on separate shelves in the medication room.
- One hospital created a chart comparing generic and trade names and attached it to the narcotics box.
- One hospital created a chart depicting and comparing all vials and ampules stocked to identify look-alike drugs.

11 Automate Carefully

Automation can reduce errors that occur in repetitive tasks or in tasks requiring attention to details. Automation becomes hazardous, however, when it leads the operator to feel less responsibility for the task or to become less expert in carrying it out should the equipment fail. Automation can multiply an error if the error is made in generating inputs to the system. It can also render the effects of an error invisible until it is too late to correct.

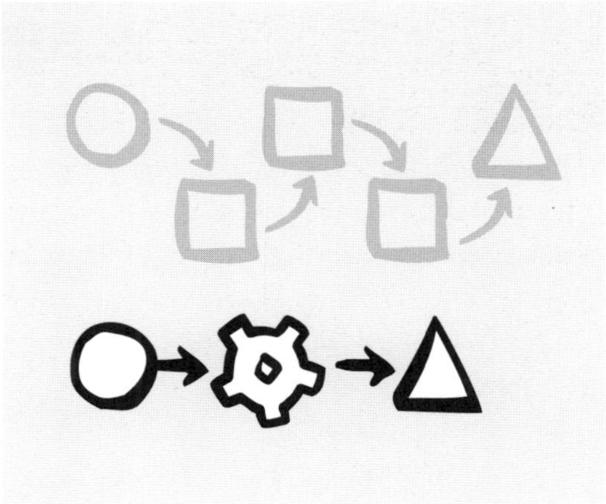

Changes that lead to careful automation:

- Use computerized order entry systems with range checks and override capacity.
- Use robotic dispensing systems in the pharmacy.
- Train staff to double check the automation regularly; this will keep their skill levels high and reinforce the idea that all systems must be monitored.
- Use bar code technology to identify drugs.

Examples:

- Many organizations use automated drug-dispensing machines on their units to reduce handoffs and make the dispensing process quicker.
- Hospitals regularly use infusion pumps to regulate the flow of IV fluids. Well-designed pumps give information about the cause of an alarm, have moderate sensitivity, and prevent free flow when the unit is turned off.

Change Concepts for **Organizational Change**

Improving organizational and environmental factors provides health care organizations the opportunity to make significant systems changes without having to redesign major hospital systems or necessarily use substantial additional resources. If teams work effectively, communication improves and personnel are motivated to understand errors and prevent them. Some of the redesign work happens naturally. Task and process redesign are powerful tools, but unless the organization has a culture that supports understanding and reducing errors, the effect will be minimal. The ideal approach to error prevention is coupling changes in the organization with concerted efforts to improve the medication system.

12 Optimize the Work Environment for Safety

The conditions under which people work can make them more or less error-prone. Extreme fatigue, for example, increases the likelihood of errors. Fortunately, it is possible to control several factors that increase the error rate. Particularly when the situation requires a high level of mental alertness, as in the operating room, the emergency department, and the intensive care unit, or in situations in which high-hazard substances are being handled, changing the environment can do much to prevent errors.

Changes that optimize the work environment for safety:

- Keep workloads within an acceptable range.
- Reduce unnecessary time pressure in any phase of the medication system.
- Avoid double shifts; accommodate diurnal sleep rhythms.
- Adjust the physical environment to increase light, decrease noise, and decrease clutter.
- Keep critical equipment available, in good repair, and stored in a uniform manner.
- Reduce distractions.

Examples:

- Several organizations provided quiet space for working on medications. Such distraction-free environments promote increased levels of concentration and should, therefore, reduce errors in ordering and administration.
- One hospital made sure that the unit clerks had a quiet area to transcribe orders from the physician order sheet—a good idea from a human factors perspective.
- Another hospital set up a chemotherapy ordering room with all the information needed on protocols, adequate desk space, and a telephone that did not ring in.
- Another organization, to avoid interruptions in patient care, began taking messages for nurses rather than paging them when a nonemergency call came in.
- Pharmacies often designate one person to dispense IV infusions or chemotherapy. This ensures that the person completing these high-hazard tasks has sufficient time and no interruptions.
- Although hospitals may not have enough staff to eliminate double shifts, many have implemented policies to ensure that those who are most likely to be fatigued, and thus most vulnerable to error, are given the responsibility for less acute patient care during their second shift.

13 Increase Feedback

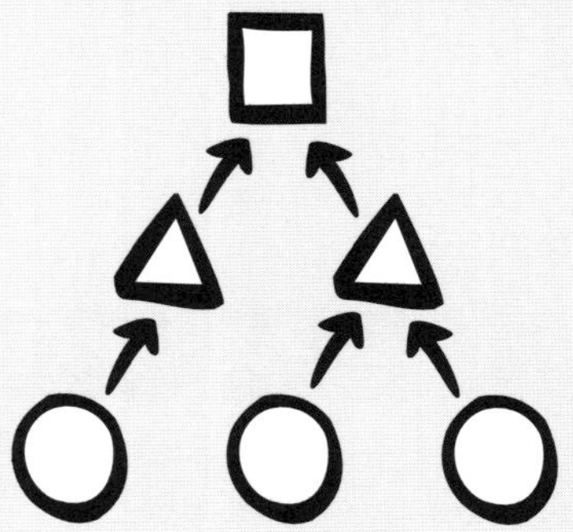

Most people want to do the right thing. As a result, they will often "self-correct" if they are aware of deficiencies that are leading to faulty performance. Similarly, knowing that what they are doing is effective boosts self-esteem and confidence, further improving performance. Providing feedback about corrective actions encourages people to identify and report errors. (One reason for low incident reporting in most hospitals is that personnel perceive that reporting has no constructive consequences.)

Finally, feedback on the effectiveness of medications, either from patient reports or from clinical information like lab results, guides timely and appropriate modification of the treatment if needed.

Changes that increase feedback:

- Use equipment that not only indicates there is a problem but also shows where the problem is.
- Monitor the effectiveness of protocols instituted and provide information to all staff demonstrating the effectiveness of protocols.
- Make staff aware of responses to reported errors.

Examples:

- Several organizations instituted heparin protocols and then monitored their effectiveness. They documented results, including reductions in the time needed to achieve therapeutic levels and the number of tests that fell within therapeutic range, and shared these results with the staff using the protocols. Such communication and follow-up encourage continued improvement of the protocol and continued enthusiasm for its use.
- Provide follow-up to error reports by letting the staff know what measures are being taken to find the causes of problems and to address those causes. One approach is to use a newsletter format that describes the error, the system problems that led to the error, and the changes made to address those problems. Presenting this information at regular staff meetings will help increase awareness of the potential for errors and create a culture that looks for system (not people) solutions to these problems.
- Staff thrive when they are able to see the results of their actions. Giving staff feedback helps them to understand the process and the quality of their work. Examples of effective feedback include the following:
  - Post a weekly summary of error reports to encourage reporting and to identify progress toward safer practice.
  - Videotape and review surgery to increase understanding of team dynamics and to identify areas for improvement in technique and process.
  - Tell the staff about actions taken to reduce errors in response to their reporting and analysis of the errors.

14 Train for Teamwork

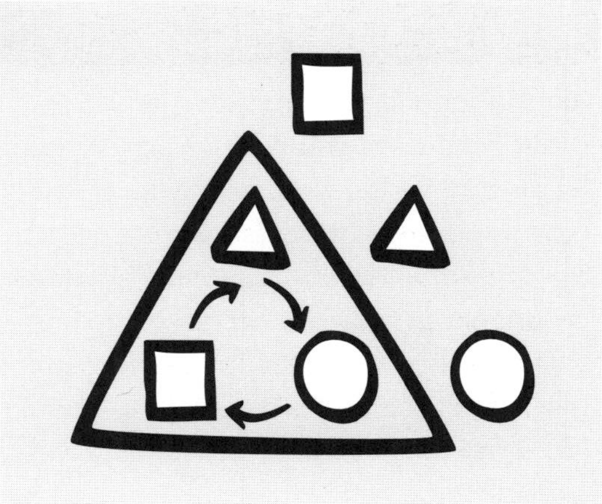

Experience from the aerospace industry demonstrates that effective teams produce fewer errors. A team that has worked together for a period of time has developed more effective communication tools and can serve as a buffer to individual errors. Training for hazardous situations prepares personnel to take the right steps under pressure.

In health care, tradition, hierarchies, and power relationships, along with inconsistent staffing and temporary staff, make achieving effective teamwork a challenge. Nevertheless, training of all personnel, along with developing a culture that expects teamwork, will greatly improve the staff's capacity to reduce errors.

Changes that support teamwork for error reduction:

- Train leaders in a nonauthoritarian style of management.
- Train workers to function as a team.
- Train workers to be interdependent as well as independent.
- Train for safety; emphasize potential hazards and methods to avoid them.
- Create stable teams to work with high-hazard substances.

Examples:

- For most organizations, it is not possible to match nurses, pharmacists, and physicians in consistent teams on the nursing units. However, consistent teams can be created in the operating room, emergency department, and some intensive care units. Working with familiar staff allows for easier communication and the ability to anticipate requests. Furthermore, consistent teams can recognize the strengths and weaknesses of each member and establish processes to compensate for any potential problems.
- Many hospitals have a chemotherapy team that works together consistently. Team members are few, all know the protocols, and their small numbers make effective communication among them much more likely. Also, these teams have well-established relationships that allow for smoother decision making. Smooth decision making, in-depth knowledge of the clinical process, and rapid, clear communication all enhance a team's ability to deal with high-hazard substances.
- Teams have simulated operating rooms, emergency departments, and Code Blue situations to give them practice working together under stressful circumstances. Simulation and role playing allow teams to practice the right skills and obtain guidance from skilled coaches without risk to the patient. These exercises decrease errors and improve team productivity.

15 Drive Out Fear

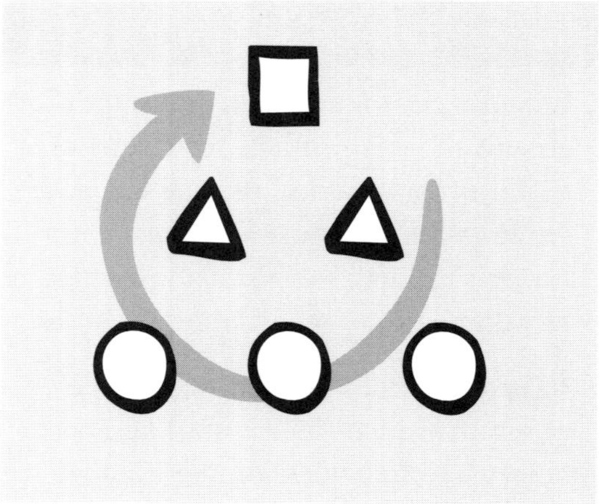

Enlisting the assistance of all health care personnel in the search for errors in work processes can prove a powerful way to reduce errors as well as to help hospital personnel understand the benefits—both personal and organizational—of learning from errors. Making personnel aware of the potential for error is not enough. Real change requires trusting that those who make errors will be dealt with in a nonpunitive manner. Staff must feel free to report errors so that the error-prone parts of the system can be understood and changed. In most health care organizations staff are reluctant to report errors because of fear of punishment. As a result, most errors are not reported, the root causes are not explored, and the opportunity to prevent the error from occurring again is lost. Physicians, in particular, do not want to increase their exposure to a malpractice suit.

The solution to this problem requires first, the decision among leadership to drive fear out of the system, and second, training leaders in nursing, pharmacy, and medicine in a supportive management style. Once senior leadership institutes a nonpunitive reporting system, staff will usually participate enthusiastically in analyzing the causes of errors and designing system changes to reduce potential errors.

Changes that drive out fear:

- Publicly reward reports of error (for example, with release time or a thank-you from the CEO).
- Establish safe havens for error reporting; for example, grant immunity from punishment.
- Establish confidential reporting of errors.
- Make error reporting easy; for example, use simple forms.
- Conduct regular small group discussions of "errors waiting to happen."
- Collect and disseminate information on common errors in the organization (for example, feed back information to clinicians).
- Display run charts to show the effects of error reduction efforts, such as compliance with protocols, reduction of nonstandard orders, or automatic dose reduction for the elderly.
- Display run charts to show increased reporting of errors.

Examples:

- Many organizations have instituted confidential error reporting systems so that anyone can report any error without fear of reprisal. The fear of punishment can seriously hamper reporting. One organization in the Collaborative found that spontaneous reporting elicited reports on only 2% of errors. With *confidential* reporting and streamlined reporting forms, the rate of error reports increased as much as twenty-fold.

  Note: Although an anonymous reporting system will increase the number of reported errors, such systems often make it impossible to find out why the error occurred. In terms of follow-up especially, a *confidential* reporting system combined with an atmosphere of trust works far better.
- Some institutions regularly present and analyze errors in the spirit of process improvement. In some cases, the person who made the error conducts the analysis and presents potential solutions to the staff. In these institutions the organizational culture promotes collegiality, group problem-solving, and open discussion of ways to improve safety.
- In an effort to understand quickly where the system is error-prone, some organizations ask small focus groups of nurses to identify the parts of the process where errors are waiting to happen. In one such session, nurses provided 50 ideas for process improvements that ranged from the storage of narcotics to faulty IV pumps. Remember: Staff members closest to the process know best where latent errors lurk. Armed with this information, teams can target certain processes for improvement.

16 Obtain Leadership Commitment

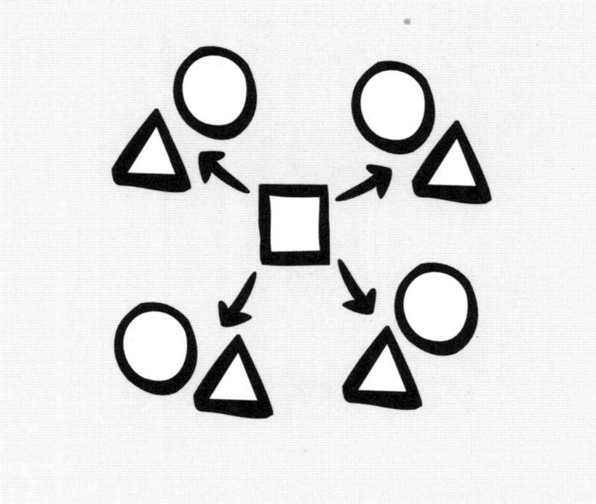

The assumption that individuals cause errors and that education and discipline will eliminate errors is common in health care and has perpetuated a system that has an alarming error rate. This assumption must change if the health care industry is to achieve greater patient safety.

System leaders must promote a system perspective, understand human error, and act to drive fear out of the system. Without the support of system leaders, error prevention will not happen.

Changes in leadership that prevent errors:

- Decrease competition and increase cooperation among staff.
- Create interdisciplinary teams.
- Publicly thank staff for reports of error.
- Commit resources to making the environment safe, establishing effective error reporting systems, improving work conditions, and providing time to analyze errors.

Examples:

- One executive sent thank-you notes to staff members who reported errors, a gesture that boosted staff morale.
- The teams that addressed adverse drug events in most hospitals represent key disciplines—pharmacy, medicine, nursing, management, quality improvement, and risk management. While in many cases the pharmacy's level of participation surpassed that of other disciplines, all team members contributed to the effort to reduce errors.
- Leadership behaviors that proved helpful to teams include the following:
  - One chief executive officer wrote an article for the health system newsletter about error reduction, highlighting the team's work.
  - Another chief executive officer made reports on adverse drug events and error reduction a top agenda item at quality council meetings and an agenda item at meetings of the Board of Trustees.
  - Several organizations allocated resources from the information systems department to assist in data collection on errors.

17 Improve Direct Communication

Communication among physicians, pharmacists, nurses, and patients is the glue that holds together the medication system. Verbal communication is faster and easier but fraught with opportunities for error. Orders should be written in such a way as to reduce possible misunderstandings. Using standard terminology and repeating back the order will help reduce errors.

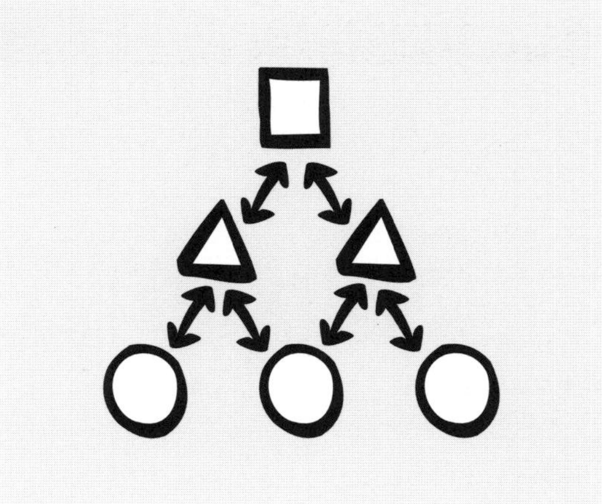

Changes that improve communication:

- Train all staff to avoid indirect and mitigated communication.
- Repeat verbal orders verbatim.
- Role-play direct communication and methods for dealing with authoritarian style.
- Provide feedback (including feedback in videotape format) about indirect and mitigated communication.

Example:

- Many organizations have established policies to reduce verbal orders or allow them only under specific circumstances because they are so prone to error. One way to minimize the risk of error is to train nursing staff and physicians to use "hear-back." When the nurse receives a verbal order, he or she repeats the order verbatim to the person who gave it, and the person giving the order must listen carefully to confirm that the order repeated is the one that was given. This skill takes practice and motivation, and so far, no organization in the Collaborative has been able to enforce such a policy.

THUS FAR IN THE GUIDE, YOU HAVE LEARNED:

Part 1 *The Model for Improvement, which can be applied to any area you want to improve.*

Part 2 *A step-by-step guide to using that model to work on reducing adverse drug events, with each of the basic steps—setting aims, forming the team, establishing measures, and developing and testing changes—illustrated with examples.*

Part 3 *A group of change concepts that can be applied in different ways throughout the medication system to reduce adverse drug events.*

Part 4

Achieving Breakthrough Improvement in Reducing Adverse Drug Events

This section provides a comprehensive guide to reducing adverse drug events by showing how organizations in the Collaborative applied the change concepts introduced in Part 3, to different parts of the medication system. Part 4 contains the following sections:

THE BASICS

THE MEDICATION SYSTEM (FLOWCHART)

Changes to Improve the **Ordering** Process

Changes to Improve the **Dispensing** Process

Changes to Improve the **Administration** Process

The Basics The first steps for error

In the long run, effective error prevention for most hospitals will require substantial redesign of their medication systems. However, in the short run, organizations can achieve substantial gains in patient safety by implementing widely accepted processes and procedures that have already been demonstrated to be effective. Most of these can be implemented promptly without prior data collection or analysis of errors, and provide a sure way to prevent or greatly reduce certain errors.

1

Enforce standardized prescribing

Many errors result from sloppy or hurried prescribing practices—abbreviating, using code symbols, or leaving out elements of the order. Well-publicized and firmly enforced prescribing rules will reduce errors.

Basic rules for standardized prescribing:

- Use the word "unit," not "u" or "U".
- Do not use the letter "Q" or "q" (QD, QID, etc.). Use "Every."
- Use leading zero (0.1 mg, not .1 mg) but not trailing zero (2 mg, not 2.0 mg).
- Include all elements of the order—dose, strength, units (metric), route, frequency, and rate.
- Use full names (preferably generic).
- Use only authorized abbreviations.
- Use metric system only.

prevention in every hospital

2

Simplify

Complexity is a cause of error. The more steps, handoffs, and communication required in a process, the greater the likelihood of error. Eliminating any of the steps in a process reduces the chances of error. Streamlining even a part of the medication system will almost always reduce errors.

Changes to simplify the process:

- Eliminate the transcription process by computerization or automatic copying of orders.
- Limit the number of possible concentrations for a drug, particularly high-hazard drugs like morphine, heparin, etc.
- Limit the types of infusion pumps to one or two.

3

Standardize multiple processes

Widely used in other industries, standardization is the simplest, most broadly applicable and effective method for reducing errors. Standardization is a form of simplification. If all personnel know and follow a single procedure or practice, they are less likely to make errors and more likely to discover errors made by others.

Candidates for standardization include:

- Doses
- Times of administration (for example, antibiotics)
- Packaging and labeling
- Storage (for example, placing medications in the same place in each unit)
- Dosing scales (for example, insulin, potassium)
- Protocols for the use and storage of potentially lethal drugs: potassium injection, insulin, lidocaine, sodium chloride injection, calcium injection, magnesium injection, chemotherapeutic agents, heparin, dextrose injection, narcotics, adrenergic agonists, theophylline

4

Use unit dosing

Unit dosing, introduced 20 or more years ago, is perhaps the most powerful change ever implemented in the medication system. It substitutes routine and repetitive pharmacist calculation and dispensing for the nonroutine process of the nurse preparing each individual medication, which is a different calculation and task each time. While somewhat more expensive than bulk dispensing and on-site preparation, unit dosing costs less overall by virtue of preventing errors in drug administration that could have far more costly results.

5

Use pharmacy-based admixture of IV medications

The error-preventive effect of pharmacy IV admixture is analogous to that of unit dosing. Both are examples of the improved efficiency and accuracy that result from specialization. IV calculations and mixing are ad hoc, on-the-spot events when performed on the nursing unit, fraught with error because they are performed occasionally and with a multitude of drugs. In a pharmacy admixture program, standardization and repetition make errors much less likely.

8

Eliminate too-long or double shifts

Fatigue degrades performance; tired workers make more errors. Health care is unique among the hazardous industries (such as aviation or nuclear power) in that this well-known fact is often ignored.

9

Use computerized drug profiling in the pharmacy

Every pharmacy should have a complete drug database for each patient against which staff can check each new prescription prior to dispensing the medication. This check system should identify therapeutic duplication, contradictory orders, and potentially harmful drug-drug interactions.

6

Use error-preventive packaging

The Food and Drug Administration (FDA) and drug manufacturers have not done all they could to ensure that pharmacists and nurses can easily tell drugs apart. "Look-alike" packages and ambiguous or unclear labels lead to errors. Pharmacies can repackage look-alikes and provide distinctive packages and labels for lethal drugs. They also can ensure that the labels on all drugs have clear, dark, large, and easy-to-read type.

7

Make allergy information available

Too often, hospitalized patients receive drugs to which they have a known allergy. Hospitals with programs that ensure that all parties—doctors, pharmacists, and nurses—have allergy information available when they need it and for each patient have substantially reduced this risk. This information should be prominently displayed on the order sheets, in the pharmacy, and on the medication administration record (MAR).

10

Institute 24-hour pharmacy service

Only pharmacists should dispense medications. Permitting nonpharmacy personnel (such as the nursing supervisor) to access the pharmacy during off hours is unwise. If there is doubt that this is a problem, ask: Would anyone sanction the reverse—a pharmacist substituting for the nurse or physician during off hours?

11

Have an effective system to monitor and report adverse drug events

Few hospitals are aware of the extent of adverse drug events because staff, fearing punishment or because the reporting system is too complex, do not report errors. When hospitals create a nonpunitive environment and encourage and reward reporting, they will begin to understand the nature and extent of their ADEs, which is the first step toward redesigning systems to reduce errors.

The Medication System

Every organization needs to implement "the basics" as the first step in reducing adverse drug events. But for most hospitals, effective error prevention will require redesign of their medication systems. The medication system in a typical hospital consists of a number of sequential actions carried out by doctors, clerks, pharmacists, technicians, and nurses. At each stage multiple factors determine whether the task will be performed without error. An error-free end result depends on error-free performance at each stage.

Unfortunately, those participating in this system tend to focus on their own part of the process and overlook the extent to which parts of the process are interrelated and the extent to which errors early in the process may cause later errors.

The flowchart is an example of a typical medication system, from ordering through dispensing and administration. Each step is annotated with some of the factors that affect the accuracy and efficiency with which the step is completed.

Most of the steps are critical control points, that is, steps where preventing errors is crucial because unchecked errors can lead to multiple errors later on. Actually, almost every stage in the medication system is a critical control point—but some are more critical than others. While no two hospitals have precisely the same system, all share some essential elements and their accompanying hazards.

Ordering

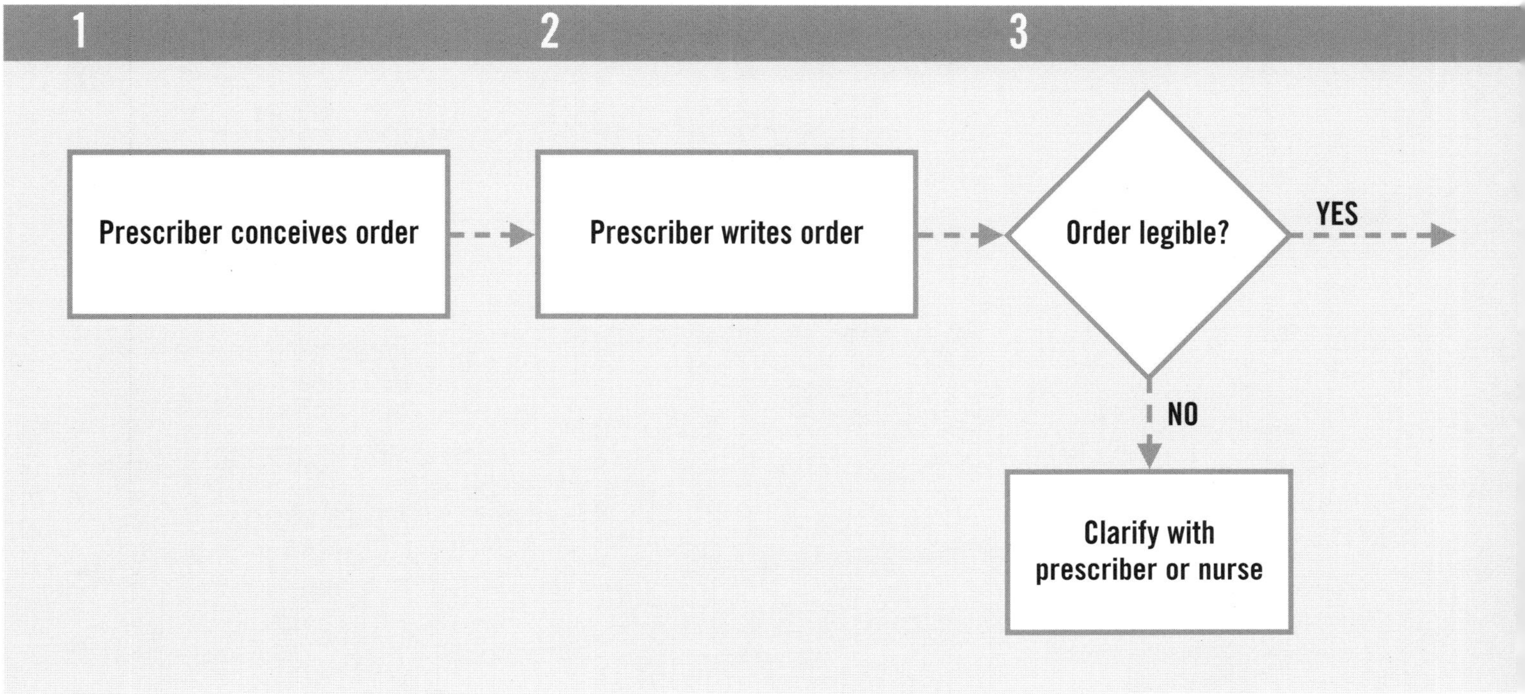

Prescriber conceives order

The key factor at this step is information: For the prescriber to make a sound decision, the system must provide the *right* information, *when* it is needed, and *where* it is needed, in an *easy-to-use* format.

Prescriber writes order

Having decided on a drug, does the prescriber write the order correctly? Too often, the answer is no. Errors at this point in the process have a cascade effect and, if not picked up early, can cause a chain of errors—by pharmacy and nursing—that can result in harm to the patient.

Here the issue is communication. Prescribers often write orders that are hard to read, nonstandard in form, and use unauthorized abbreviations. The goal is to ensure unambiguous, error-free communication.

Order legible?

How does the system deal with illegible orders? Do nurses or pharmacists inform prescribers that orders are illegible and clarify questions, or do they resolve the issue informally by guessing (and increase the potential for misinterpretation)?

Ordering (continued)

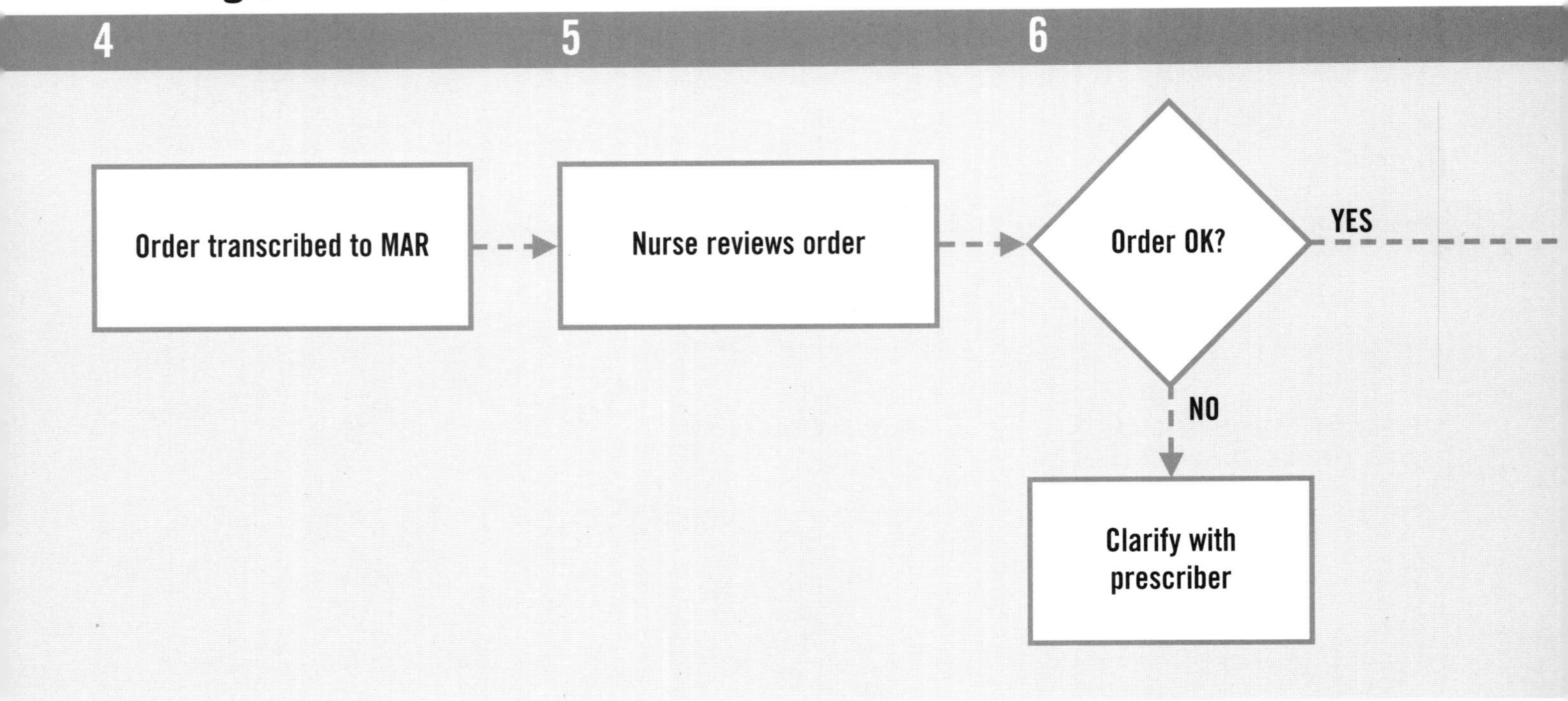

Order transcribed to MAR

This is often a clerical function with many opportunities for error. The clerk, who may not be very familiar with medications, writes in the medication administration record (MAR) what the prescriber has ordered. Both the legibility of the order and the accuracy of entering the information determine whether this handoff happens without error.

Nurse reviews order

The nurse must make sure that the order is correct: proper in form, unambiguous, and appropriate for the patient. The key to this step is the availability of information. To begin with, the nurse needs to be informed that a new order has been written. What is the system for making sure the nurse is aware of a new order? How does the system ensure that the MAR and the appropriate drug and patient information are available?

Order OK?

If there is a problem with the order, the nurse must consult with the prescriber to clarify the order.

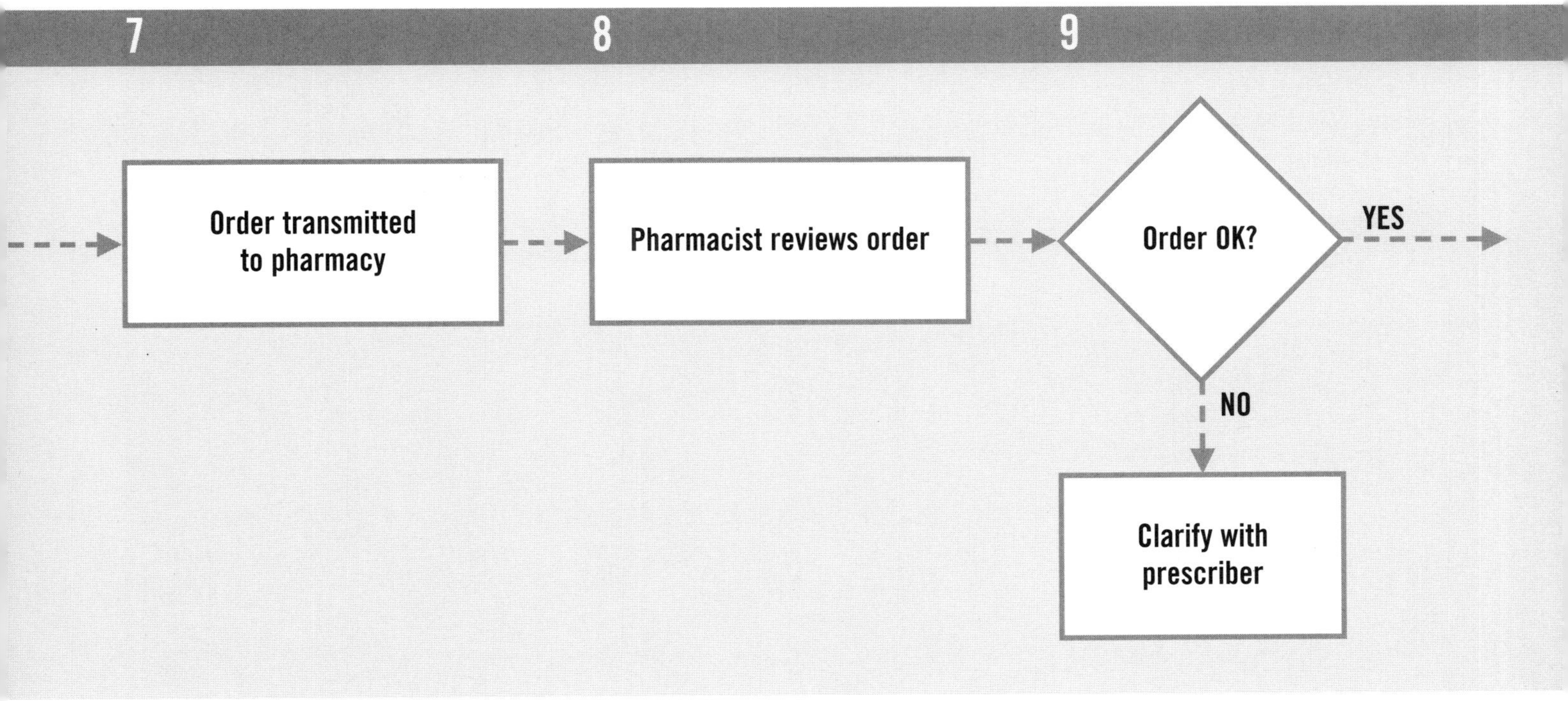

Order transmitted to pharmacy

How is the order transmitted? Whether by fax, pneumatic tube, computer, hand carried, or telephone, each method carries its own unique potential for error.

Pharmacist reviews order

Again, the key is the availability of information. The pharmacist must have the information he or she needs, including:

- Drug information, with dose, form, and compatibility
- Patient information, including age, height, and weight
- Clinical judgment: Is this an appropriate drug for this patient?
- Therapeutic duplication: Is the patient receiving another medication with similar effect?

Order OK?

If the order is unclear, the pharmacist must intervene and consult with the prescriber to clarify the order. Pharmacists frequently intercept prescribing errors, but the goal is to have a system that works so well that such interception becomes virtually unnecessary.

Dispensing

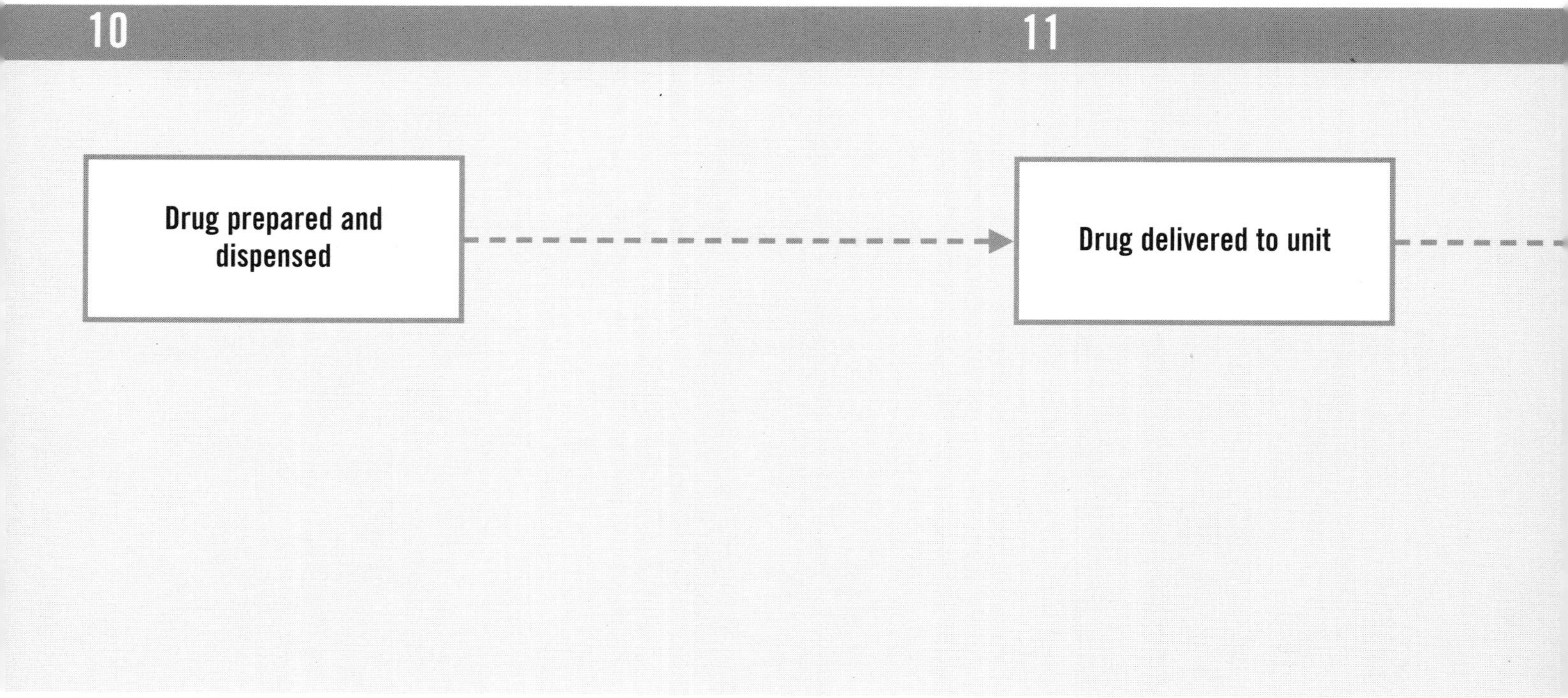

Drug prepared and dispensed

Before an order arrives, two issues must be resolved:
- Drug purchasing: Are drugs provided in appropriate forms and packages and with labeling that minimizes errors?
- Drug storage: Are "look-alike" or "sound-alike" drugs stored separately so that they cannot easily be confused?

The following factors relate specifically to the dispensing function. Here, careful reading, accuracy, and vigilance are important.

To ensure accuracy, the system must address the following:
- Is it the right drug (no mistakes due to look-alikes or sound-alikes)?
- Is the drug appropriate for the patient?
- Did the pharmacist screen for drug-drug interaction, therapeutic duplication, appropriate dosing (age and weight check or body surface area), route, and frequency?
- Are the dose and amount calculated correctly?
- Is the dose prepared correctly?
- Is the packaging unique and not easily confused with another drug?
- Is the labeling clear, including drug identity, dose, and patient identity?

Drug delivered to unit

This handoff has a high potential for error. To ensure accuracy, the system must address the following:

- Is the drug delivered to the right unit, to the right patient, at the right time?
- Are "look-alike" drugs stored separately in the unit?
- If drugs are delivered to a dispensing machine, what procedures are in place to prevent errors?
- If drugs are delivered in unit dose carts, what ensures that the cart-filling process was correct?

Administration

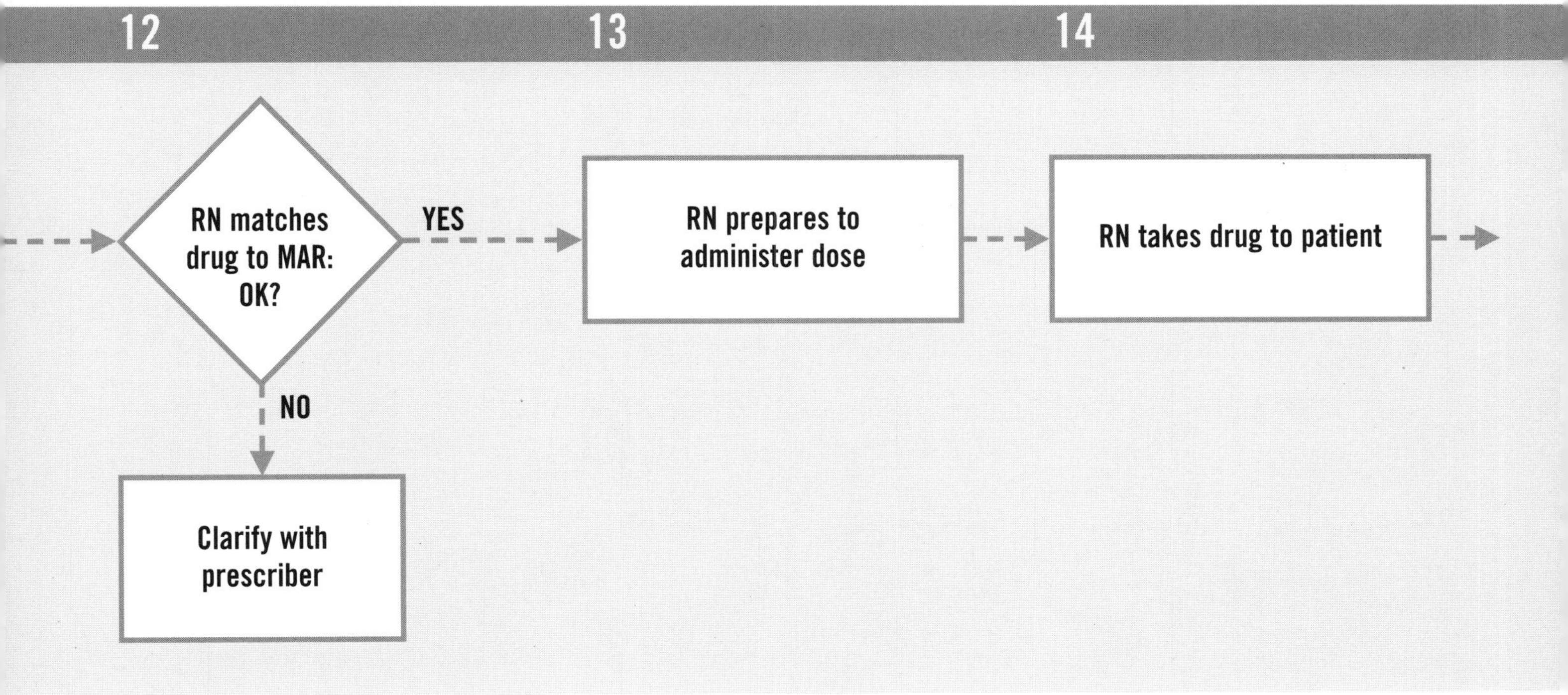

RN matches drug to MAR

Verification by the nurse is vital for the system to ensure the drug dose is given as prescribed and as recorded in the medication administration record. And conversely, the nurse must check that the MAR is accurate and up to date regarding drugs given, times, and other details.

RN prepares to administer dose

The goal of this step is to achieve the "Five Rights": the right drug gets to the right patient in the right dose at the right time by the right route.

To ensure accuracy, the system must answer the following:

- Are monitoring data available when and where needed?
- Are there protocols that apply? Does the dose fit?
- Is the dispensing machine used properly? Does it increase or decrease errors?
- Is unit dosing used?
- If unit dosing is not used, then how are calculation, counting, and measuring accuracy ensured?

RN takes drug to patient

This process may not be as straightforward as it seems:

- Are medications prepared a long distance away?
- Will there be distractions along the way?
- If the patient is not in the room, when can the dose be given?

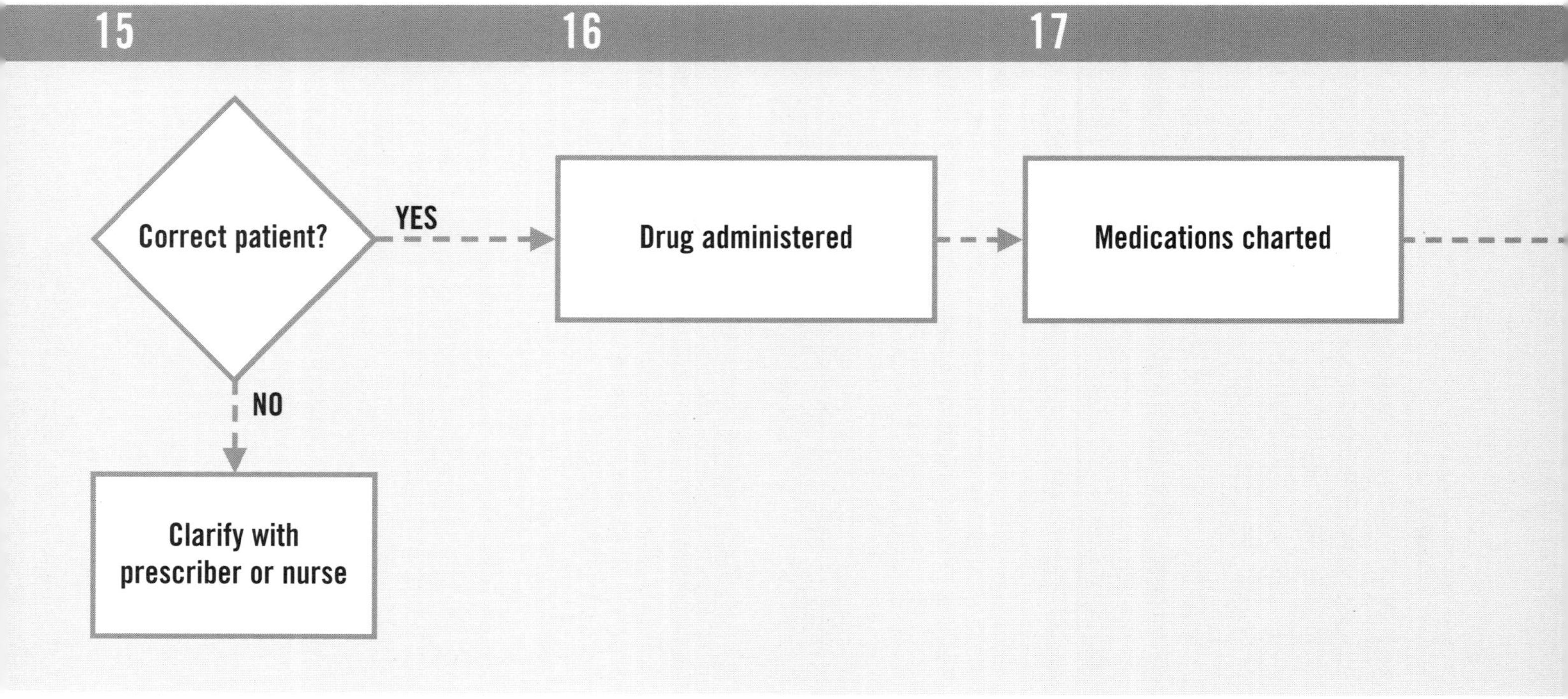

Correct patient?

Is there a fool-proof system for ensuring that the medication is given to the correct patient?

Drug administered

Each route has its own risks. Parenteral use, in particular, can result in many errors. A host of technical factors can combine to cause errors, including IV equipment malfunction or pump failures.

Self-administration has some advantages, but may pose additional problems.

Medications charted

Are all medications charted in one place so that anyone—doctors, pharmacists, nurses—can easily find out whether a patient has received a dose, or are there multiple records that potentially lead to errors and confusion? Are medications charted correctly?

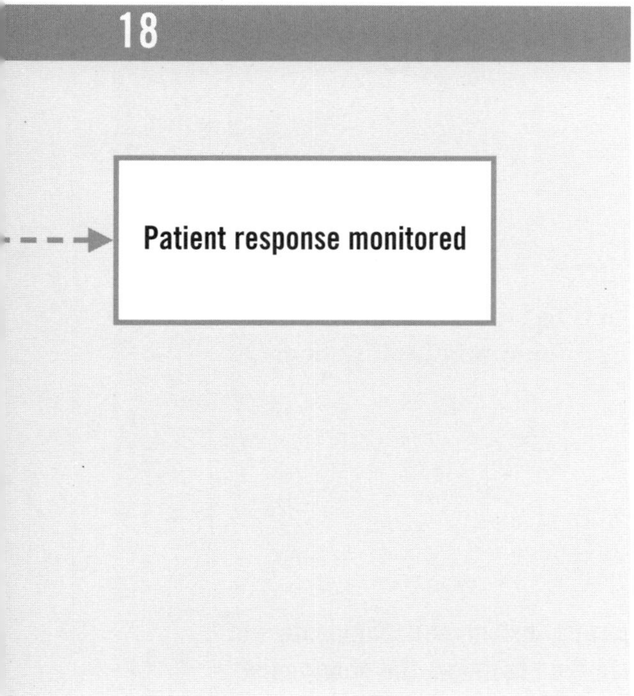

Patient response monitored

Is the necessary information about a patient's response to medication available on a chart when needed? Are procedures in place to initiate a change if the response is not as expected?

IMPROVING THE MEDICATION SYSTEM

Each major process in the medication system—ordering, dispensing, and administration—has its own unique opportunities for error. However, a few key change concepts have been found to be particularly useful in redesigning all three processes to improve patient safety.

For each major process in the medication system, the charts on pages 92–118 indicate the following:

- **Change concepts that are useful in redesigning the process**
- **Problems in applying each change concept**
- **Useful process changes**
- **Examples of process changes tested by organizations either before or during the Collaborative**
- **Resources**

  This symbol indicates that a resource developed by an organization in the Collaborative is included at the end of Part 4.

Changes to Improve the Ordering Process

Change Concept

Reduce Reliance on Memory

Ordering Problems

- There are too many drugs and too many facts to be remembered.
- When prescribers rely on memory, they forget important details about drugs or patients.

Useful Process Changes

- **Use computerized prescriber order entry.**
- **Use preprinted orders.**
- **Use guided dose algorithms.**
- **Check dose ranges.**
- **Use protocols for hazardous drugs (chemotherapy, insulin, anticoagulants, etc.).**
- **Make accurate allergy information available to the physician, the pharmacist, and the nurse.**
- **Use an automatic dose reduction plan.**

Examples of Process Changes Tested

Antibiotic Order Form
(pp. 119–120)
Children's Hospital, Boston

Use preprinted orders.

Using dosing algorithms reduces the need to rely on memory. Dosing algorithms have been used successfully in the administration of antibiotics, chemotherapeutics, heparin, and parenteral nutrition. Many algorithms can be printed on order sheets so that a physician writing an order can insert patient information into the formula that is already printed and calculate the dose. Eliminating the need to remember multiple formulas makes dosing far more reliable.

Tested and implemented by:

Allegheny General Hospital
Bay Medical Center
The Cambridge Hospital
Cedars-Sinai Medical Center
Children's Hospital, Boston
Dartmouth-Hitchcock Medical Center
Deaconess-Nashoba Hospital
Fairview Health System
Garden City Hospital
Kaiser Foundation Health Plan, Inc.
Kaweah Delta Health Care District
Kimball Medical Center
Latrobe Area Hospital
Lucile Salter Packard Children's Hospital at Stanford
Northwest Covenant Medical Center
Paoli Memorial Hospital
Pontiac Osteopathic Hospital Medical Center
Promina Gwinnett Health System
The Valley Hospital

Creatinine Clearance Protocol (p. 121)
Fairview Health System

Use an automatic dose reduction plan.

Elderly patients and patients with renal failure need to receive substantially lower doses of many medications than those generally prescribed for adults. Physicians frequently forget to prescribe lower doses for these patients. One hospital instituted a program in which the pharmacist automatically reduces doses as needed for elderly patients and those with renal failure, thus virtually eliminating overdosing in these patients.

Tested and implemented by:

Fairview Health System
Kaweah Delta Health Care District
Promina Gwinnett Health System

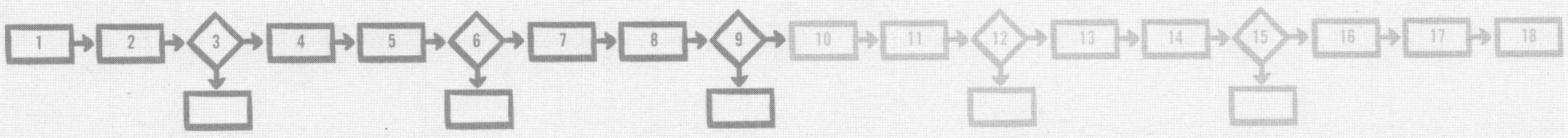

Change Concept

Simplify

Ordering Problems

- The large number of drugs increases the likelihood of error.
- The need for transcribing orders introduces an additional opportunity for error.

Useful Process Changes

- **Limit the number of drugs in the formulary.**
- **Limit the number of dose options.**
- **Use protocols for hazardous drugs.**
- **Eliminate transcription.**

Examples of Process Changes Tested

Limit the number of drugs in the formulary.

Many highly toxic drugs or drugs likely to be used incorrectly have little therapeutic advantage over other less hazardous drugs designed to treat the same disorders. One hospital removed these hazardous drugs from the formulary, thus eliminating hundreds of potential adverse drug events per year.

Tested and implemented by:

Dartmouth-Hitchcock Medical Center
Deaconess-Nashoba Hospital
Fairview Health System
Kaweah Delta Health Care District
Morton Plant Mease Health Care
Northwest Covenant Medical Center
Promina Gwinnett Health System

Change Concept

Standardize

Ordering Problems

- Stylistic practices, such as individual differences in the use of terminology, use of improper abbreviations, and failure to follow rules continue to be tolerated.
- Physicians use multiple "sliding scales" for insulin.

Useful Process Changes

- **Use standard usage rules (for example, "unit" not "u"; leading not trailing zeroes).**
- **Use abbreviations sparingly; use standard abbreviations only.**
- **Use standard measures (metric).**
- **Use preprinted orders.**
- **Reject illegible orders.**

Examples of Process Changes Tested

Adult Medication Order Guidelines (pp. 122–123)
Dartmouth-Hitchcock Medical Center

Reject nonstandard orders.

Many organizations set standards for prescribing practices, including rules for appropriate abbreviations and notations. They notified medical staff in staff meetings, sent letters to all, put the information in newsletters, and placed a laminated copy of the standards on all charts. All orders were clarified and filled promptly, but after three weeks, physicians still using nonstandard notation received in the mail their nonstandard orders accompanied by a "pink slip." This process proved very effective, and the percentage of nonstandard or illegible orders received in the pharmacy dropped by 60%.

Tested and implemented by:

Bay Medical Center
Cedars-Sinai Medical Center
Dartmouth-Hitchcock Medical Center
Deaconess-Nashoba Hospital
Grand View Hospital
Kaiser Foundation Health Plan, Inc.
Morton Plant Mease Health Care
Munson Medical Center
Paoli Memorial Hospital
Pontiac Osteopathic Hospital Medical Center
Promina Gwinnett Health System
The Valley Hospital

Change Concept

Use Constraints and Forcing Functions

Ordering
Problems

- Excessively hazardous drugs are ordered when safer substitutes are available.
- Many ordering processes permit ordering of toxic or lethal doses.

Useful Process Changes

- **Use computerized order entry.**
- **Make high-hazard drugs and doses unavailable for use.**
- **Allow certain drugs to be used only by protocol.**

Examples of Process Changes Tested

Use computerized order entry.

Most computerized order entry systems are programmed so that medications have dose range checks based on the age, height, and weight of patients, as well as screens for allergies. The prescriber cannot specify a dose that is improper for the patient. A more sophisticated system can calculate dosages for the prescriber, given the medication, its indication, and the height, weight, and age of the patient. Of course, most of these systems allow the user to override the computer, but to do so requires some effort—which often allows the prescriber time to reflect on the correct dose.

Tested and implemented by:

Bay Medical Center
Children's Hospital of Philadelphia
Dana-Farber Cancer Institute
Maine Medical Center

Change Concept

Use Protocols and Checklists Wisely

Ordering Problems

- Complicated medication routines, such as those used for anticoagulation and for chemotherapy, frequently lead to errors.

Useful Process Changes

- **Use protocols for hazardous drugs.**
- **Use preprinted orders.**

Examples of Process Changes Tested

Orders for Chemotherapy
(pp. 124–125)
Fairview Health System

Use protocols for hazardous drugs.

Organizations that administer chemotherapy use a checklist to initiate the infusion. The checklist includes such items as patient identifiers; double-checks on the medication, route, and dose; checks for lab values that might indicate a different approach to treatment; and the status of the infusion device and intravenous access line. The nurse administering the chemotherapy also goes through the checklist carefully before beginning the infusion.

Tested and implemented by:

Allegheny General Hospital
Bay Medical Center
The Cambridge Hospital
Children's Hospital of Philadelphia
Dana-Farber Cancer Institute
Deaconess-Nashoba Hospital
Deaconess-Waltham Hospital
Fairview Health System
Garden City Hospital
Latrobe Area Hospital
Lucile Salter Packard Children's Hospital at Stanford
Maine Medical Center
Northwest Covenant Medical Center
Pontiac Osteopathic Hospital Medical Center
Promina Gwinnett Health System
The Valley Hospital

Change Concept

Improve Access to Information

Ordering
Problems

- Medical records and nursing charts do not make information easily available. Few are on-line.
- Drug information is not easily available at the time it is needed.
- Communication among multiple caregivers is often incomplete.

Useful Process Changes

- **Use a computerized medical record.**
- **Use computerized order entry.**
- **Have a pharmacist make rounds with doctors and nurses.**
- **Have a pharmacist available on the unit rather than in the pharmacy.**
- **Make protocols available at order entry.**
- **Provide for effective recovery and display of allergy information.**
- **Provide for effective feedback of lab findings.**

Examples of Process Changes Tested

Have a pharmacist make rounds with doctors and nurses.

Several organizations have begun to include a clinical pharmacist on the nursing units. Having pharmacists available when physicians are writing orders (during rounds) allows for a dialogue between physicians and pharmacists concerning specific medications and makes it easier to get the order right the first time. This also prevents the delay in ordering that occurs when an incorrect order goes to the pharmacy before the error is identified and corrected, usually requiring an additional call to the physician.

Figure 4.1 shows the increase in the number of days between medication interventions that occurred at one hospital when a pharmacist began participating in ICU rounds in October 1996. When this pilot test stopped in November, the interventions again became more frequent.

Tested and implemented by:

The Cambridge Hospital
Dana-Farber Cancer Institute
Dartmouth-Hitchcock Medical Center
Deaconess-Waltham Hospital
Kaweah Delta Health Care District
Northwest Covenant Medical Center
Pontiac Osteopathic Hospital Medical Center
The Valley Hospital

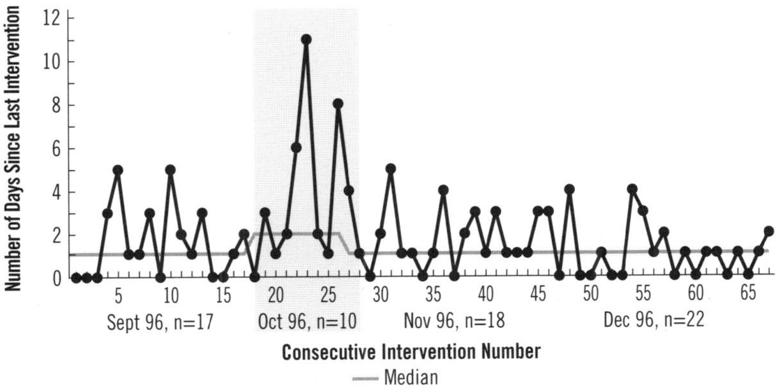

Figure 4.1
Increase in Days Between Medication Interventions (Longer Is Better)

The Cambridge Hospital
Cambridge, MA

Changes to Improve the Dispensing Process

Change Concept	Reduce Reliance on Memory
Dispensing Problems	• Drug and patient information is too extensive and complicated to remember. • Look-alike and sound-alike drugs are difficult to distinguish.
Useful Process Changes	**• Use computerized order entry.** **• Use computer profiling of patient data.** **• Use computerized drug information.** **• Use computerized alerts.** **• Use preprinted orders.** **• Use robotic dispensing.** **• Bar-code drugs.** **• Label boldly and clearly.** **• Print recommended rate of administration on label.**

Examples of Process Changes Tested

Use computer profiling of patient data.

Many pharmacies use computers to profile patients' medications and monitor utilization. These systems use a checking program to identify drug-drug interactions. When a new prescription is entered for a patient, the program searches available patient information and identifies contraindications for use of that drug.

Tested and implemented by:

The Cambridge Hospital
Children's Hospital, Boston
Kaiser Foundation Health Plan, Inc.
Latrobe Area Hospital
Maine Medical Center
Morton Plant Mease Health Care
Northwest Covenant Medical Center
Promina Gwinnett Health System
St. Marys Hospital Medical Center

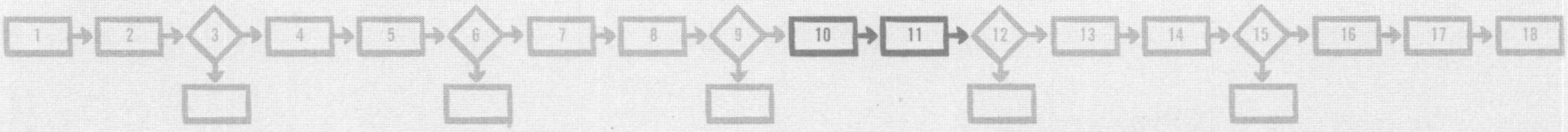

Change Concept

Simplify

Dispensing Problems

- Multiple dosage forms increase the opportunity for error.
- Multiple steps in the dispensing process increase the likelihood of error.

Useful Process Changes

- **Limit the choice of drugs.**
- **Limit the doses for each drug.**
- **Limit the number of administration times.**
- **Institute a pharmacy IV admixture program.**
- **Repackage drugs to eliminate look-alikes.**
- **Allow automatic drug dispensing on the nursing unit.**

Examples of Process Changes Tested

Limit the doses for each drug.

Several organizations have limited the concentrations of heparin solutions available on the nursing units to one. Nurses report fewer near misses—times when they almost used the wrong strength.

Most hospital pharmacies are able to identify the two or three IV solutions that are used most often and how much of these solutions is used each day. In several organizations, the pharmacy mixed a stock of these solutions in a batch each day so that during the press of a busy day only a few had to be mixed to order. There was occasional waste when solutions expired, but teams believed that the errors prevented by doing the admixture on the slower-paced night shift more than compensated for this cost.

Tested and implemented by:

Allegheny General Hospital
Children's Hospital, Boston
Deaconess-Nashoba Hospital
Dartmouth-Hitchcock Medical Center
Fairview Health System
Northwest Covenant Medical Center
Promina Gwinnett Health System

Change Concept

Standardize

Dispensing Problems

- Manufacturers do not provide standardized products or packaging.
- Pharmacists sometimes have idiosyncratic practices.

Useful Process Changes

- **Standardize the following: doses, dosing times, storage locations, concentrations, packaging, labels, delivery times.**
- **Institute an IV admixture program.**
- **Use protocols for hazardous drugs.**
- **Conduct a systematic review of every order.**

Examples of Process Changes Tested

Standardize doses.

Restricting the number of dose choices reduces errors. Not only is there less for everyone to remember, but when doctors, pharmacists, and nurses become accustomed to the standard doses, they instantly recognize when an error has been made.

Tested and implemented by:

Allegheny General Hospital
Bay Medical Center
Children's Hospital, Boston
Children's Hospital of Philadelphia
Dartmouth-Hitchcock Medical Center
Fairview Health System
Good Samaritan Regional Health Center
Grand View Hospital
Lucile Salter Packard Children's Hospital at Stanford
Maine Medical Center
Morton Plant Mease Health Care
Paoli Memorial Hospital
Promina Gwinnett Health System
The Valley Hospital

Standardize packaging and labels.

One organization stocked two concentrations of morphine sulfate in identical cartridges. In order to prevent wrong-dose errors, the pharmacy labeled the higher concentration cartridge with bright orange tape. This extra packaging step prevented mix-ups in administering the morphine and averted cases of overdose.

Tested and implemented by:

Allegheny General Hospital
Bay Medical Center
Children's Hospital, Boston
Dartmouth-Hitchcock Medical Center
Deaconess-Nashoba Hospital
Grand View Hospital
Kaiser Foundation Health Plan, Inc.
Morton Plant Mease Health Care
Promina Gwinnett Health System
The Valley Hospital

Change Concept

Use Constraints and Forcing Functions

Dispensing Problems

- Stylistic practices exist in the pharmacy; different pharmacists dispense and label medications differently.
- Medication orders can be processed without the pharmacy knowing a patient's clinical conditions (for example, allergies or renal failure).
- Toxic drugs can be ordered in excessive doses.

Useful Process Changes

- **Program the computer not to process an order unless key information has been entered.**
- **Dispense epidural medications only in unique spinal syringes.**
- **Remove hazardous drugs of limited value from the formulary.**
- **Use automatic dose reduction for the elderly and patients with renal failure.**

Examples of Process Changes Tested

Program the computer not to process an order unless key information has been entered.

An effective way to eliminate errors is to program the pharmacy computer to require entry of certain critical information (such as drug allergies, height, weight, date of birth) before an order for medication can be processed. The responsibility for obtaining these data still rests with the nurse, but this change ensures a fail-safe check before any medication is dispensed.

Tested and implemented by:

Bay Medical Center
Dana-Farber Cancer Institute
Garden City Hospital
Grand View Hospital
The Valley Hospital

Change Concept

Use Protocols and Checklists Wisely

Dispensing Problems

- Complicated processes are difficult to remember.
- Variation in the use of hazardous drugs increases the likelihood of error.

Useful Process Changes

- **Use protocols for hazardous drugs.**
- **Require double check by a second person for hazardous drugs.**

Examples of Process Changes Tested

Require second checks for hazardous drugs.

Checklists and preprinted protocols are especially useful in dealing with hazardous drugs where errors can potentially be fatal.

In the pharmacy, most chemotherpeutics and total parenteral nutrition (TPN) solutions are double checked by a second pharmacist before dispensing.

Tested and implemented by:

Bay Medical Center
Cedars-Sinai Medical Center
Children's Hospital, Boston
Dana-Farber Cancer Institute
Deaconess-Nashoba Hospital
Deaconess-Waltham Hospital
Morton Plant Mease Health Care
Northwest Covenant Medical Center
Promina Gwinnett Health System
The Valley Hospital

Change Concept

Improve Access to Information

Dispensing Problems

- Important patient information (for example, presence of allergies and laboratory data) is not always sent to the pharmacy.

Useful Process Changes

- **Use computerized order entry.**
- **Use computer profiling of patient data.**
- **Use computerized drug information.**
- **Make the formulary available on-line.**
- **Use computerized alerts.**
- **Use preprinted orders.**
- **Print IV administration guidelines and compatibility charts.**
- **Use on-line laboratory data.**
- **Include critical information on drug labels.**

Examples of Process Changes Tested

Use computerized alerts.

Program pharmacy computers to deliver a warning when an abnormal laboratory finding (such as a very high PT or PTT) is obtained, as well as when the patient is taking another medication that is incompatible with a new drug being ordered.

Tested and implemented by:

Bay Medical Center
The Cambridge Hospital
Children's Hospital, Boston
Dana-Farber Cancer Institute
Northwest Covenant Medical Center
Promina Gwinnett Health System

Change Concept

Decrease Reliance on Vigilance

Dispensing Problems

- Look-alike and sound-alike drugs increase the chance of errors.
- Pharmacists may fail to intercept out-of-range doses.
- Errors will occur when only one person is responsible for preventing them.

Useful Process Changes

- **Institute automatic, daily monitoring of doses of toxic drugs (for example, chemotherapy).**
- **Eliminate look-alike drugs. Repackage as needed.**
- **Store look-alike drugs separately.**
- **Develop a system to differentiate sound-alike drugs.**
- **Enlist the patient and family in vigilance tasks.**

Examples of Process Changes Tested

Institute automatic, daily monitoring of doses of toxic drugs (for example, chemotherapy).

Have another observer monitor the use of toxic drugs. One hospital used a clinical pharmacist to monitor daily the use of high-hazard substances on specific units. Heparin, aminoglycosides, chemotherapeutics, and experimental drugs are examples of the types of medications that require increased attention.

Tested and implemented by:

Dana-Farber Cancer Institute
Fairview Health System
Promina Gwinnett Health System

Eliminate look-alike drugs. Repackage as needed.

One organization stocked two concentrations of morphine sulfate in identical cartridges. To reduce wrong-dose errors, the pharmacy labeled the higher concentration cartridge with bright orange tape. (See "Standardize packaging and labels" on p. 100.)

Tested and implemented by:

Bay Medical Center
Children's Hospital, Boston
Dartmouth-Hitchcock Medical Center
Deaconess-Nashoba Hospital
Fairview Health System
Garden City Hospital
Grand View Hospital
Kaweah Delta Health Care District
Munson Medical Center
Northwest Covenant Medical Center
Promina Gwinnett Health System

Change Concept

Reduce Handoffs

Dispensing Problems

- Multiple participants—pharmacists, technicians, clerks, and others—increase the chance of error.

Useful Process Changes

- **Use computerized order entry.**
- **Use computerized order transfer.**
- **Use a satellite pharmacy.**
- **Use a computerized medication administration record (MAR).**
- **Use robotic dispensing.**
- **Use unit dosing.**
- **Use automatic dispensing.**

Examples of Process Changes Tested

Use a satellite pharmacy.

Decentralization of pharmacy functions increases the ease of communication and reduces the number of people involved in each drug handoff. In addition, the principle of "going where the action is" not only makes the pharmacist more accessible, but enhances the job satisfaction of some pharmacists by making them more personally involved in the patient care process.

Tested and implemented by:

Children's Hospital, Boston
Promina Gwinnett Health System

Changes to Improve the Administration

Change Concept

Reduce Reliance on Memory

Administration Problems

- There are too many drugs and too many facts to remember. Nurses may forget patients' drug allergies.
- On-time administration of medications depends on the nurse's memory.

Useful Process Changes

- **Make allergy information readily available.**
- **Use patient allergy color-coded wristbands.**
- **Partner with the patient.**
- **Make drug information readily available.**
- **Bar code drugs.**
- **Use timers or reminder systems.**
- **Use IV guidelines.**
- **Use protocols for hazardous drugs.**
- **Use protocols for epidural medications.**
- **Use guidelines for the use of infusion pumps.**
- **Reduce variation in equipment and supplies.**

Examples of Process Changes Tested

Partner with the patient.

Enlist the assistance of conscious and cooperative patients by asking them to double check what medications they are getting and when. In one organization, the patients received a list of their medications daily. When the nurse came to administer medications, the nurse reviewed the list with the patients. This offered both a double check and an opportunity to educate the patient. Using this method prevented many errors, and the patients liked being involved in their care as well.

Tested and implemented by:

Promina Gwinnett Health System

The Valley Hospital

Use timers or reminder systems.

In one organization, the IV antibiotics often "ran out" and were not switched back to the main IV bag because the nurse, busy with other patients, forgot to change the bag. The solution: Nurses hung small digital timers on the doors of patients' rooms to remind them when to change specific IV piggyback medications. If the patient's nurse was not nearby, someone else would hear the alarm and notify the nurse, who could then make the appropriate change.

Tested and implemented by:

Dartmouth-Hitchcock Medical Center

Promina Gwinnett Health System

Process

Examples of Process Changes Tested (continued)

Use IV guidelines.

One organization wanted to ensure the accuracy of cardiovascular drip rates for NICU patients, concerned that the process of calculating drips under urgent conditions was prone to error. To prevent miscalculations, the team in the NICU developed a guideline for mixing the solutions and setting the drip rate to maintain the proper dose and fluid volume per hour.

Cardiac Drip Worksheet
(pp. 126–127)
Lucile Salter Packard Children's Hospital at Stanford

Tested and implemented by:

Children's Hospital, Boston
Deaconess-Nashoba Hospital
Deaconess-Waltham Hospital
Kimball Medical Center
Northwest Covenant Medical Center
Pontiac Osteopathic Hospital Medical Center

Change Concept — Simplify

Administration Problems

- The need for the nurse to mix medications provides an opportunity for error.
- Some hospitals use multiple types of infusion pumps.
- Multiple participants, multiple drugs, and multiple dose strengths make administration complex and susceptible to error.

Useful Process Changes

- **Limit the following: choice of drugs, access to the medication room, doses for each drug, number of administration times.**
- **Institute a pharmacy IV admixture program.**
- **Institute automatic drug dispensing on the nursing unit.**
- **Reduce the number of protocols for hazardous drugs (for example, KCl, insulin, anticoagulants, chemotherapy).**
- **Use unit dosing.**
- **Have a single record for entry of medications.**
- **Use standard equipment with simple instructions and a convenient user interface.**

Examples of Process Changes Tested

Limit the number of administration times.

Many organizations have shifted to once-per-day aminoglycoside doses, thus preventing the need to adjust the dose throughout the day based on blood levels from the lab.

Tested and implemented by:

Deaconess-Nashoba Hospital
Deaconess-Waltham Hospital
Morton Plant Mease Health Care
Northwest Covenant Medical Center
Promina Gwinnett Health System
St. Marys Hospital Medical Center

Institute a pharmacy IV admixture program.

In most organizations, the pharmacy places additives in IV solutions. Removing the task of calculating and mixing additives such as KCl from nursing staff simplifies the administration process for the nurses. The pharmacy is better organized to carry out this process, providing the required accuracy and a distraction-free environment. The properly mixed solution comes from pharmacy when needed, and the nurse need only verify correctness and calculate the flow rate (perhaps using an IV drip rate "cheat sheet"). Purchasing premixed solutions from the manufacturer reduces the risk of errors even further.

Tested and implemented by:

Children's Hospital, Boston
Grand View Hospital
Promina Gwinnett Health System

Examples of Process Changes Tested (continued)

Reduce the number of protocols for hazardous drugs (for example, potassium chloride, insulin, anticoagulants, chemotherapy).

Many organizations have simplified their work by restricting the number of protocols for the same medication. When nurses have three or four heparin protocols, it is easier for them to confuse which protocol is being used. Using only one protocol for deep vein thrombosis prophylaxis and one for treatment of embolism helps staff remember what is required.

Tested and implemented by:

Children's Hospital of Philadelphia
Dartmouth-Hitchcock Medical Center
Fairview Health System
Garden City Hospital
Good Samaritan Regional Health Center
Maine Medical Center

Use unit dosing.

In most organizations, medications arrive at the floor ready to be packaged and administered specifically to each patient. The pharmacy fills a drawer for each patient with single-dose packages of the medications ordered for the patient for the day and brings the drawer to the unit. The nurse need not prepare the medications from a vast floor stock, a task that requires making calculations and drawing up or mixing the medications. The task is simplified: the nurse finds the medication ordered in the drawer, verifies the correctness (right dose, drug, time, patient, and route), and administers it to the patient.

Tested and implemented by:

Children's Hospital, Boston
Deaconess-Nashoba Hospital
Promina Gwinnett Health System

Use equipment with simple instructions and a convenient user interface.

Hospitals frequently use infusion pumps to regulate the flow of IV fluids. Nursing staff rely on the accuracy and good working order of these pumps. Pumps that frequently deliver false alarms are annoying, and the nursing staff may respond by ignoring the alarms or turning them off. Select pumps that give information about the cause for the alarm, have moderate sensitivity, and prevent free flow when the unit is turned off. Also, stock only one or two types of pumps per nursing unit.

Change Concept

Standardize

Administration Problems

- For certain drugs, ordered doses vary widely.
- Administration times for ordered drugs vary widely.
- Physicians use multiple dosing scales for insulin, heparin, and other medications.
- Complex drug regimens are difficult to follow.

Useful Process Changes

- **Standardize the following: doses, administration times, delivery times, storage locations, concentrations, infusion pumps**
- **Institute an IV admixture program.**
- **Use preprinted orders.**
- **Use protocols for hazardous drugs.**
- **Use protocols for epidural infusion.**

Examples of Process Changes Tested

How to Stagger Antibiotics to Get Them on Standard Times (p. 128)
St. Marys Hospital Medical Center

Standardize administration times.

One organization established a protocol for administration of prophylactic, preoperative antibiotics that require that the first dose be given in the holding area just before wheeling the patient into the operating room. Thus, they reduced the interval from first dose to incision time to 60 minutes—a reduction of 66% from previous levels.

Tested and implemented by:

Children's Hospital of Philadelphia
Deaconess-Nashoba Hospital
Deaconess-Waltham Hospital
Kimball Medical Center
Lucile Salter Packard Children's Hospital at Stanford
Morton Plant Mease Health Care
Northwest Covenant Medical Center
Promina Gwinnett Health System
St. Marys Hospital Medical Center

Standardize storage locations.

Every medication room in a hospital is laid out in the same way and medications are stored in the same place. One organization decided to store the two concentrations of IV heparin on separate shelves in the medication room. Storing look-alike bags side-by-side had been a case of wrong-dose errors waiting to happen. After changing the location of the higher-dose bag and notifying nurses of the change, the number of near misses (taking the wrong concentration off the shelf) decreased.

Tested and implemented by:

Bay Medical Center
The Cambridge Hospital
Dartmouth-Hitchcock Medical Center
Deaconess-Nashoba Hospital
Grand View Hospital
Munson Medical Center

Examples of Process Changes Tested (continued)

Sliding-Scale Insulin Protocol for Adults
(p. 129)
Garden City Hospital

Use protocols for hazardous drugs.

Many organizations used insulin sliding-scales and chemotherapy, potassium replacement, and other protocols. The protocols educated staff such that everyone knew what was expected. Completing the task the same way each time eliminated confusion among staff as to what would be the next step or who was responsible. In addition, protocols eliminated the need for time-consuming ad hoc communication with the prescriber about lab results and dosing.

Tested and implemented by:

Allegheny General Hospital
The Cambridge Hospital
Children's Hospital of Philadelphia
Deaconess-Nashoba Hospital
Deaconess-Waltham Hospital
Fairview Health System
Garden City Hospital
Lucile Salter Packard Children's Hospital at Stanford
Maine Medical Center
Northwest Covenant Medical Center
Pontiac Osteopathic Hospital Medical Center
Promina Gwinnett Health System

Change Concept

Use Constraints and Forcing Functions

Administration Problems

- Availability of concentrated potassium chloride permits accidental fatal injection.
- Similar fittings permit accidental IV injection of gastrostomy feeding solution.
- Certain drugs (for example, KCl, insulin) can easily be fatal if the wrong dose is accidentally given.

Useful Process Changes

- **Remove hazardous drugs from the nursing unit (for example, concentrated KCl).**
- **Use special fittings to prevent the mismatch of enteral and parenteral medications to the wrong route.**
- **Limit access to the medication room.**

Examples of Process Changes Tested

Remove hazardous drugs from the nursing unit (for example, concentrated KCl).

Many organizations removed concentrated potassium from floor stock, thus forcing the admixture process to the pharmacy. This constraint prevents the accidental infusion of concentrated potassium (which causes eight to twelve deaths annually in U.S. hospitals) and also decreases the likelihood of inaccurate dosing due to admixture mistakes on the nursing units.

Tested and implemented by:

Allegheny General Hospital
Dartmouth-Hitchcock Medical Center
Deaconess-Nashoba Hospital
Deaconess-Waltham Hospital
Fairview Health System
Garden City Hospital
Grand View Hospital
Kaiser Foundation Health Plan, Inc.
Kaweah Delta Health Care District
Morton Plant Mease Health Care
Munson Medical Center
Northwest Covenant Medical Center
Paoli Memorial Hospital
Pontiac Osteopathic Hospital Medical Center
Promina Gwinnett Health System
The Valley Hospital

Change Concept

Use Protocols and Checklists Wisely

Administration Problems

- Multiple dosing schedules for hazardous drugs increase the potential for error.
- On-time administration of medications (for example, preoperative antibiotics) depends on nurse memory.
- Complex processes are difficult to remember accurately.
- Some regimens (for example, chemotherapy) must be carried out precisely.

Useful Process Changes

- **Use protocols for hazardous drugs.**
- **Use protocols for epidural drugs.**
- **Use protocols for preoperative antibiotics.**
- **Coordinate insulin dosing with labs and meals.**
- **Use double check systems for blood products and high-hazard substances.**

Examples of Process Changes Tested

Heparin Protocol Dosing Order Sheet (p. 130)
Latrobe Area Hospital

Use protocols for hazardous drugs.

By establishing one weight-based heparin protocol for prophylaxis, organizations eliminated the constant phoning and dosage adjustment that occurs in the absence of the protocol. The nursing staff learn just one protocol and become familiar with it, which, in turn, allows them to speed up the steps required to respond to lab results. As a result of one organization's work, the average time required to reach a therapeutic level dropped from more than 24 hours to less than 8 hours, and the number of dosage adjustments decreased as well.

Tested and implemented by:

Children's Hospital, Boston
Garden City Hospital
Latrobe Area Hospital
Northwest Covenant Medical Center
Promina Gwinnett Health System
The Valley Hospital

Change Concept

Improve Access to Information

Administration Problems

- Medical records and nursing charts are not organized to make information easily available. Few are on-line.
- Drug and patient information is not readily available when and where nurses need it.
- There are too many drugs and too many facts for nurses to remember.

Useful Process Changes

- **Make allergy information prominently available on the medication administration record (MAR).**
- **Provide a pharmacist on the unit.**
- **Make computerized drug information easily accessible.**
- **Make patient clinical and lab information available on-line.**
- **Display protocols in the medication room.**
- **Have patients wear color-coded allergy wristbands.**
- **Partner with patients about drug names, doses, and times.**
- **Locate the MAR at the bedside.**
- **Place commonly used information where it is needed.**
- **Post generic/trade name "translation" charts.**

Examples of Process Changes Tested

Have patients wear color-coded allergy wristbands.

One organization instituted a red identification wristband for patients with drug allergies. The red color prompted the nursing staff to recheck allergies prior to giving any medications, thus preventing the patient from receiving the wrong medication.

Tested and implemented by:

Bay Medical Center
Pontiac Osteopathic Hospital Medical Center

Locate the medication administration record (MAR) at the bedside.

One organization moved the medications and the medication administration record to the bedside. With this information available at the point of administration, it was much easier to see what the patient needed, and omissions, wrong doses, and wrong-drug errors were prevented. This system required extra steps to update medication administration records when orders changed, but the errors averted by having information available at the bedside more than compensated for the extra work.

Tested and implemented by:

Morton Plant Mease Health Care
Promina Gwinnett Health System

Examples of Process Changes Tested (continued)

Medication Administration Times for Food/Drug Interactions (pp. 131–132)
Methodist Hospital/
HealthSystem Minnesota

Place commonly used information where it is needed.

Nursing staff cannot reliably recall all the necessary information concerning protocols, drug interactions, trade and generic names, and other facts. To address this problem, many organizations placed easy-to-read laminated information sheets or cards where they are needed. Dosing protocols are printed on laminated cards that clinicians can keep in their lab coat pockets. A listing of times that medications need to be given in order to avoid negative interactions with food is posted on the medication cart. IV drip rate calculation sheets are hung on IV pumps. Such "cheat sheets" serve to make information available at the point of use.

Tested and implemented by:

- The Cambridge Hospital
- Children's Hospital, Boston
- Deaconess-Nashoba Hospital
- Deaconess-Waltham Hospital
- Good Samaritan Regional Health Center
- Grand View Hospital
- Kaiser Foundation Health Plan, Inc.
- Pontiac Osteopathic Hospital Medical Center
- St. Marys Hospital Medical Center

Post generic/trade name "translation" charts.

One hospital was concerned about sound-alike and look-alike narcotics in the narcotics cabinet, as well as confusion of trade and generic names. The team put together a generic/trade name chart and attached it to the narcotics box. As a result, nurses could correctly identify the right medication, regardless of whether the ordering physician used a trade or generic name, and wrong-drug errors decreased.

Tested and implemented by:

- Deaconess-Nashoba Hospital
- Fairview Health System
- Grand View Hospital
- Morton Plant Mease Health Care
- Northwest Covenant Medical Center
- Promina Gwinnett Health System

Change Concept

Decrease Reliance on Vigilance

Administration Problems

- Fatigue, overwork, complexity of tasks, and responsibility for multiple patients make it difficult for nurses to maintain vigilance.

Useful Process Changes

- **Remove high-hazard medications from the nursing unit.**
- **Use automatic drug dose checking.**
- **Use checklists.**
- **Use premixed IV bags.**
- **Use a double check system for hazardous drugs.**
- **Eliminate look-alike drugs.**
- **Use distinctive, clear labels.**
- **Use targeted monitoring for hazardous drugs.**

Examples of Process Changes Tested

Use a double check system for hazardous drugs.

Many organizations use a double check system for administering blood products and insulin. The nurse administering the medication shows another nurse the order and the dose and explains how it was calculated. This procedure, while cumbersome, can be extended to apply to other high-hazard drugs such as narcotics, chemotherapy, and heparin. While the risk is that the double checks will be cursory, if done with care they can detect errors.

Tested and implemented by:

Bay Medical Center
The Cambridge Hospital
Cedars-Sinai Medical Center
Children's Hospital, Boston
Dana-Farber Cancer Institute
Deaconess-Nashoba Hospital
Deaconess-Waltham Hospital
Northwest Covenant Medical Center
Promina Gwinnett Health System
The Valley Hospital

Narcotic Flowsheet
(p. 133)
Kaweah Delta Health Care District

Use targeted monitoring for hazardous drugs.

Monitors that track the therapeutic effects and side effects of specific drugs reduce reliance on vigilance. One organization noticed excessive narcotics doses and instituted routine monitoring of respiration rate every hour for patients on narcotics. The use of antidotes for narcotic overdose decreased to near zero.

Monitoring the electrocardiogram for any patient on cardiac active drugs and monitoring blood pressure electronically for patients on vasopressors are other examples of targeted monitoring.

Tested and implemented by:

Kaweah Delta Health Care District

Change Concept

Reduce Handoffs

Administration Problems

- Late delivery of medications from the pharmacy can result in omissions and late administration.
- Multiple staff working with medications increase handoffs on the nursing unit.

Useful Process Changes

- **Use unit dosing.**
- **Use automatic drug-dispensing machines.**
- **Use patient self-administration of drugs.**
- **Use patient partnering.**

Examples of Process Changes Tested

Use automatic drug-dispensing machines.

Automatic drug-dispensing machines stock up to 70% of the most commonly used medications on each nursing unit. A copy of the physician's order is sent to the pharmacy for review. If the order is appropriate, the pharmacist enters the order into the pharmacy system. Through an interface, the order is shared with the automatic drug-dispensing machine, and the nurse may access the medication directly from the machine. These systems help to prevent the administration of a medication to a patient with a known allergy and minimize confusion over brand and generic names. However, the systems have their own potential for errors—they must be filled correctly, and the nurse must still select the correct medication.

Tested and implemented by:

Bay Medical Center
Latrobe Area Hospital
Morton Plant Mease Health Care
Pontiac Osteopathic Hospital Medical Center
Promina Gwinnett Health System
The Valley Hospital

Use patient self-administration of drugs.

In some hospitals, capable patients are allowed or even encouraged to administer their own medications. Particularly for pain control or medications taken over a long period of time (such as insulin or cardiac medications), patients can assume continuing self-care. This reduces the need for both pharmacy and nursing to be involved in the administration process and allows patients some control over their medication regimen. It also eliminates another opportunity for error—handoffs from pharmacy to nursing to patient.

Tested and implemented by:

Promina Gwinnett Health System

Resources

The Medication System

Antibiotic Order Form

Children's Hospital, Boston

Creatinine Clearance Protocol

Fairview Health System

Adult Medication Order Guidelines

Dartmouth-Hitchcock Medical Center

Orders for Chemotherapy

Fairview Health System

Cardiac Drip Worksheet

Lucile Salter Packard Children's Hospital at Stanford

How to Stagger Antibiotics to Get Them on Standard Times

St. Marys Hospital Medical Center

Sliding-Scale Insulin Protocol for Adults

Garden City Hospital

Heparin Protocol Dosing Order Sheet

Latrobe Area Hospital

Medication Administration Times for Food/Drug Interactions

Methodist Hospital/HealthSystem Minnesota

Narcotic Flowsheet

Kaweah Delta Health Care District

CHILDREN'S HOSPITAL, BOSTON

Antibiotic Order Form

Use this form to document all new antibiotic orders. A new form must be used for changes or additions. Rewrites every 7 days.

Patient Weight ____ kilograms

Allergies ____ ☐ None known

Routine Surgical Prophylaxis: Single dose recommended to be administered at time of incision.

Circle to Order	Fill in: mg dose	Recommended Dose	Route	Interval	Circle # of Doses
cefazolin		30 mg/kg per **Dose**	IV	q8h	1 2 3 doses

Routine Antibiotic Orders: Circle choice, fill in dose, duration and circle interval, route.

Circle Antibiotic	Unit Dose (Fill in: mg)	Daily Dose Range (divided by administration frequency for unit dose)	Circle Route	Circle Interval every "x" hours	Fill in Duration of Rx (Max 7 days)
amphotericin B		0.25–1 (mg/kg/day)	IV	24	___ days *or* ___ doses
ampicillin		100–400 (mg/kg/day)	IV IM	6	___ days *or* ___ doses
amp/sulbactam		100–200 AMP (mg/kg/day)	IV IM	6	___ days *or* ___ doses
cefazolin		50–100 (mg/kg/day)	IV IM	8	___ days *or* ___ doses
clindamycin		15–40 (mg/kg/day)	IV IM	8	___ days *or* ___ doses
gentamicin		4.5–7.5 (mg/kg/day)	IV IM	8 12 24	___ days *or* ___ doses
metronidazole		30 (mg/kg/day)	IV PO	6	___ days *or* ___ doses
oxacillin		150–200 (mg/kg/day)	IV IM	4 6	___ days *or* ___ doses
piperacillin		200–300 (CF300–500) (mg/kg/day)	IV IM	6	___ days *or* ___ doses
tobramycin		4.5–7.5 (CF6–10) (mg/kg/day)	IV IM	8 12 24	___ days *or* ___ doses
vancomycin		40–60 (mg/kg/day)	IV	8 12	___ days *or* ___ doses

OTHER UNRESTRICTED ANTIBIOTICS	Unit Dose (Fill in: mg)	Circle Route	Interval (Fill in)	Duration of Rx (Fill in: Max 7 days)
1.		IV IM PO	Every ___ hours	___ days *or* ___ doses
2.		IV IM PO	Every ___ hours	___ days *or* ___ doses

Restricted Antibiotic Orders: Describe intended use and provide required information.

☐ ***Preapproved indications:*** *(Refer to directions on form back.)* ***Important: Automatic stop order at 72 hours.*** Some restricted antibiotics may be used for up to 72 hours while cultures are pending. Look up the code for preapproved indications from table on reverse side of this form. Place the code after the drug name in the order box. Example: cefotaxime (2B)

☐ ***All other use of restricted antimicrobials: (Requires ID approval.)*** Indication: ____________

Fill in name of ID physician approving use: ________________________________

RESTRICTED ANTIBIOTICS (CODE) (List code if preapproved indication.)	Unit Dose (Fill in mg)	Circle Route	Interval (Fill in)	Duration of Rx (Fill in: Max 7 days)
1. ( )		IV IM PO	Every ___ hours	___ days *or* ___ doses
2. ( )		IV IM PO	Every ___ hours	___ days *or* ___ doses

Physician's signature ____________________ Date __/__/__ Time ______ Beeper __________

RN transcribing order ____________________ Date __/__/__ Time ______ Beeper __________

RN verifying transcription ____________________ Date __/__/__ Time ______ Beeper __________

CHILDREN'S HOSPITAL, BOSTON

Antibiotic Order Form (continued)

The restricted antibiotics may be used for listed indications without prior infectious disease approval. Only drugs and indications listed below are preapproved. All other use of restricted antibiotics, antifungals, and antivirals must be explicitly approved by infectious diseases prior to use.

Restricted Antibiotic (dose range)	Route	Interval	Preapproved Indications ➔ *(Copy number/letter code to front page)*
amikacin 15–22.5 mg/kg/day	IV/IM	q8h	No preapproved indications: Call infectious Diseases.
aztreonam 90–120 mg/kg/day (CF150–200)	IV	q6h or q8h	1A: Substitute for other beta-lactam antibiotics to provide gram-negative coverage if patient allergic to penicillin/cephalosporin. 1B: Substitute for aminoglycosides for gram-negative coverage in patients with or at high risk for renal insufficiency or hearing loss. 1C: Cystic fibrosis only if piperacillin or ceftazidime not appropriate.
cefotaxime 100–200 mg/kg/day	IV	q6h or q8h	2A: R/O sepsis in newly admitted patient (not nosocomial r/o sepsis). 2B: Meningitis, probable bacterial (with vancomycin if gram-positive). 2C: R/O sepsis if penicillin-resistant pneumococcus is likely (or vancomycin).
ceftazidime (CF150–200)	IV	q8h	3A: Cystic fibrosis only when piperacillin not appropriate (allergy, resistance). 3B: Empiric treatment for fever and neutropenia when piperacillin + gentamicin not appropriate due to allergy.
ceftriaxone 50–75 mg/kg/day	IV/IM	q24h	4A: One dose for early discharge from hospital. 4B One dose IM for temporary IV access problem.
ciprofloxacin 10–15 mg/kg/day	IV, PO	q12h	5A: Cystic fibrosis only if piperacillin or ceftazidime not appropriate.
imipenem 60–100 mg/kg/day	IV	q6h	6A: Cystic fibrosis only if piperacillin or ceftazidime not appropriate.
piperacillin/tazobactam 200–300 Pip mg/kg/day	IV	q6h	7A: Appendicitis—Note: q8h interval (preapproved for full 7-day course). 7B: Cystic fibrosis if pseudomonas and staph coverage needed (add additional piperacillin to reach total piperacillin dose of 300–500 mg/kg/day). 7C: Fever and neutropenia per Clinical Practice Guideline (duration to 7 days).
vancomycin (not restricted) 40–60 mg/kg/day	IV/PO	q8h	Vancomycin is not restricted. Guidelines for empiric use: Do not use vancomycin for empiric therapy of suspected CVL infection, post op wound infection, C. difficile diarrhea, or fever and neutropenia unless patient is critically ill. Use alternative abx until cultures confirm need for vanco.
Antivirals/Antifungals			
acyclovir 750–1500 mg/m²/day	IV	q8h	8A: Per approved protocol. Oral acyclovir is not restricted. Switch to PO form as soon as feasible.
ganciclovir 7.5–10 mg/kg/day	IV	q12h	9A: Per approved protocol
fluconazole 3–6 mg/kg/day	IV/PO	qd	10A: Per approved protocol
itraconazole 3–5 mg/kg/day	PO	qd	11A: Per approved protocol

Antibiotic Unit Doses Available from the Pharmacy

Dosing Groups	Available Doses (All orders should be in these increments)
All penicillins and cephalosporins, aztreonam, erythromycin, imipenem	50, 100, 150, 200, 250, 300, 400, 500, 750 mg: 1, 1.25, 1.5, 1.75, 2, 2.5, 3, 3.5, 4 gm etc.
clindamycin	50, 100, 150, 300, 450, 600, 750, 900 mg
gentamicin, tobramycin	1–6 mg by 0.25 mg increments; 7, 8, 9, 10, 12, 14, 16, 18, 20, 25, 30, 35, 40, 45, 50, 60, 70, 80, 90, 100 mg etc.
acyclovir, chloramphenicol, vancomycin	10–100 mg by 10 mg increments; 125–250 by 25 mg increments; 250–800 mg by 50 increments; 900, 1000 mg

General Dosing Rule: If the calculated dose (mg/kg/dose) is in the lower third of the increment, round **down**. If the calculated dose is in the upper two-thirds of the increment, round **up**.

FAIRVIEW HEALTH SYSTEM

Creatinine Clearance Protocol

Drug	Usual Dosage	30–50 mL/min	10–30 mL/min	<10 mL/min	Comments
acyclovir (IV)HSV	5 mg/kg q8h	q12h	q24h	q48h	Consult MD prior to dosage adjustment
acyclovir VSV	10 mg/kg q8h	q12h	q24h	q48h	Consult MD prior to dosage adjustment
allopurinol	300 mg qd	200 mg qd	100 mg qd	100 mg qod	
ampicillin/ sulbactam	1.5–3 g q6–12h	unchanged	q12h	q24h	
aztreonam	500–2000 mg q6–12h	unchanged	50%	25%	
cefazolin	500–2000 mg q8h	q12h	q12h	q24h	
cefotaxime	1–2 g q6–8h	unchanged	q12h	q24h	
cefotetan	1–2 g q12h	unchanged	q24h	q48h	
ceftazidime mild/mod	1 g q8–12h	q12h	q24h	500 mg q24h1	

DARTMOUTH-HITCHCOCK MEDICAL CENTER

Adult Medication Order Guidelines

1. All medication orders must be complete. A complete medication order includes:
   - Medication name
   - Dose
   - Route
   - Frequency
   - Date order written
   - Ordering provider's signature
   - Printed name or pager number of ordering provider
2. If the medication order is time sensitive (STAT, ASAP), the **time** the order is written must be included. Use "STAT" or "ASAP" when an order is time sensitive. Do **not** use "now."
3. Generic names are preferable, but the use of trade (brand) names is acceptable in two circumstances:
   (a) Combination products containing two or more drugs within one formulation (e.g., Bactrim DS Percocet)
   (b) Extended or sustained release formulations must be indicated with the name of the medication (e.g., Procan SR 500 mg OR Cardizem CD 120 mg).
4. Do **not** abbreviate medication names.
5. An order cannot be changed once it has been transcribed. It must be **rewritten**.

Legibility and Completeness of Medication Orders:

Medication orders that are illegible, unclear, or incompletely written will not be carried out until rewritten or clarified in writing. The individual who wrote the original order will be contacted. If that person is unavailable, the covering provider will be contacted.

Do (acceptable)	***Don't (not acceptable)***
Write out "microgram" or "mcg"*	Don't abbreviate: "μg"*
Write out "units"*	Don't abbreviate: "u" or "U"*
Write out "days" or "doses"	Don't abbreviate: "d" or "D"
Use a leading "0" (for example: 0.2 mg)	Don't use trailing "0" (for example: 2.0 mg)

* "μg" "u" "U" as abbreviations have led to dosing errors; these are no longer acceptable. Other metric units may be abbreviated.

Some common reasons why medication orders are unclear or incomplete:

1. Injectable formulation of medication must be ordered by dosage, not volume, for example: potassium phosphate 15 mmol (**not** 15 mL vial).

2. The use of "prn" must be accompanied by a frequency and/or indication, for example: q 6h prn; and prn loose stool max 8 tablets/24 hr (**not just** prn).

DARTMOUTH-HITCHCOCK MEDICAL CENTER

Adult Medication Order Guidelines (continued)

Verbal Orders:

Anyone taking a verbal order will write the order in the same manner as described above and be held responsible for rewriting or clarifying the order as needed. The individual taking a verbal order must write and read back the order as written to the prescriber. The verbal order must be co-signed by a physician.

Reference Sources:

The following reference sources are available to clinicians:

American Hospitals Formulary Services: Drug Information

Physicians' Desk Reference

Electronic resources (being developed)

In addition, pharmacists are available for consultation. Please contact the Pharmacy at ext. XXXX.

Approved by:
ADE Core Team
April 24, 1997

FAIRVIEW HEALTH SYSTEM

Orders for Chemotherapy

Today's Date ____________ Date of Admission ____________

Patient ____________ Height ________ Weight ________ BSA _____

1. Labs
   - ☐ Draw the following labs:
   - ☐ CBC
   - ☐ Lytes
   - ☐ Creatinine
   - ☐ SMA-12
   - ☐ Other
   - ☐ Call office for faxed results.
   - ☐ Call for lab results before initiating chemotherapy.
   - ☐ Proceed with chemotherapy if WBC> ________, platelet count > _______ and creatinine < _______.
   - ☐ Proceed with chemotherapy if lab values are within normal limits.

☐ Labs done in office: WBC _______ Hgb _______ creatinine _______

2. IV: ☐ D5 1/2 NS with 20 mEq KCl at ____________ mL/hr

☐ Standard Dosing ☐ High Dose Regimen

☐ Research Protocol ☐ CCOP ☐ Other

☐ Other Protocol: Source ____________ Tumor ____________

Drug	Dose	Route	Frequency	Special Instructions
	_____ mg _____ mg/m2 _____ units Other _______	☐ IV push ☐ IV over 24 hours ☐ IV over ____ hours ☐ Subcutaneous ☐ Oral ☐ Other _________	☐ One-time dose on _____ ☐ Daily for _________ days ☐ q ___ hours for ___ doses ☐ On day numbers _______ ☐ Other ______________	
	_____ mg _____ mg/m2 _____ units Other _______	☐ IV push ☐ IV over 24 hours ☐ IV over ____ hours ☐ Subcutaneous ☐ Oral ☐ Other _________	☐ One-time dose on _____ ☐ Daily for _________ days ☐ q ___ hours for ___ doses ☐ On day numbers _______ ☐ Other ______________	
	_____ mg _____ mg/m2 _____ units Other _______	☐ IV push ☐ IV over 24 hours ☐ IV over ____ hours ☐ Subcutaneous ☐ Oral ☐ Other _________	☐ One-time dose on _____ ☐ Daily for _________ days ☐ q ___ hours for ___ doses ☐ On day numbers _______ ☐ Other ______________	

FAIRVIEW HEALTH SYSTEM

Orders for Chemotherapy (continued)

Drug	Dose	Route	Frequency	Special Instructions
	_____ mg _____ mg/m2 _____ units Other _______	☐ IV push ☐ IV over 24 hours ☐ IV over ____ hours ☐ Subcutaneous ☐ Oral ☐ Other _________	☐ One-time dose on _____ ☐ Daily for __________ days ☐ q ___ hours for ___ doses ☐ On day numbers _______ ☐ Other ________________	
	_____ mg _____ mg/m2 _____ units Other _______	☐ IV push ☐ IV over 24 hours ☐ IV over ____ hours ☐ Subcutaneous ☐ Oral ☐ Other _________	☐ One-time dose on _____ ☐ Daily for __________ days ☐ q ___ hours for ___ doses ☐ On day numbers _______ ☐ Other ________________	

Antiemetics (prophylactics):

Start 30 min before chemotherapy:

Give every day of chemotherapy or _______________

_____ granisetron 0.01 mg/kg IV (not to exceed 1 mg)

_____ granisetron 1 mg po q12h x _____ doses

_____ ondansetron ☐ 10 mg ☐ 30 mg IV

_____ dexamethasone _____ mg IV

_____ prochlorperazine 10 mg IV or PO

_____ other ________________________________

Antiemetics (rescue):

_____ lorazepam 0.5–2 mg IV or PO q4h prn

_____ prochlorperazine 10 mg IV or PO q4h prn

_____ ondansetron 10 mg IV q4h prn

_____ other ________________________________

Follow paclitaxel or cisplatin routines (see separate page). Check here to omit ☐.

Give test dose prior to bleomycin or asparaginase. Check here to omit ☐.

Other instructions ____

____

Readmission date ____________ Physician's signature ______________________

Cardiac Drip Worksheet

Name Baby NICU

Acct # 1234567 Sex F

Unit # 1234567 Patient Location SW

Medication	Amount to Add	Stock Concentration	Med. Vol. to Add	Total Vol. in D5W:
alprostadil	1020 mcg	500 mcg/mL =	2.04 mL	QS to 50 mL
dopamine	102 mg	40 mg/mL =	2.55 mL	QS to 50 mL
dobutamine	102 mg	12.5 mg/mL =	8.16 mL	QS to 50 mL
epinephrine	1.02 mg	1 mg/mL =	1.02 mL	QS to 50 mL
esmolol	1020 mg	250 mg/mL =	4.08 mL	QS to 50 mL
isoproterenol	1.02 mg	0.2 mg/mL =	5.10 mL	QS to 50 mL
milrinone	1.02 mg	1 mg/mL =	1.02 mL	QS to 50 mL
nitroglycerin	20.4 mg	5 mg/mL =	4.08 mL	QS to 50 mL
nitroprusside*	10.2 mg	10 mg/mL =	1.02 mL	QS to 50 mL

Total Fluid Intake: 60 mL/kg/day
80 mL/kg/day
100 mL/kg/day

*Nitroprusside: Dissolve 50 mg vial in 5 mL D5W; then dilute as above.

Drips will be made in 60 mL syringes.

LUCILE SALTER PACKARD CHILDREN'S HOSPITAL AT STANFORD

Date report run 9/28/96
User name Rx
DOB 9/18/96
WT.(kg) 3.4

Final Dose Equivalence	Dose Range	Final Drip Concentration
1 mL/h = 100 ng/kg/min	25–100 ng/kg/min	0.0204 mg/mL
1 mL/h = 10 mcg/kg/min	2–10 mcg/kg/min	2.04 mg/mL
1 mL/h = 10 mcg/kg/min	2–12 mcg/kg/min	2.04 mg/mL
1 mL/h = 100 ng/kg/min	20–200 ng/kg/min	0.02 mg/mL
1 mL/h = 100 mcg/kg/min	50–200 mcg/kg/min	20.4 mg/mL
1 mL/h = 100 ng/kg/min	20–200 ng/kg/min	0.0204 mg/mL
1 mL/h = 0.100 mcg/kg/min	0.375–0.75 mcg/kg/min	0.0204 mg/mL
1 mL/h = 2 mcg/kg/min	0.5–2 mcg/kg/min	0.408 mg/mL
1 mL/h = 1 mcg/kg/min	0.5–2 mcg/kg/min	0.204 mg/mL

ST. MARYS HOSPITAL MEDICAL CENTER

How to Stagger Antibiotics to Get Them on Standard Times

Time Next Dose(s) Due per Antibiotic Interval

Time 1st IV Dose Hung	**q 6h** 0600–1200–1800–2400	**q 8h** 0600–1400–2200	**q 12h** 0800–2000	**q 24h**
2400	0600	0700–1400	1000–2000	Time
0100	0600	0700–1400	1000–2000	assigned
0200	0700–1200	0800–1400	1100–2000	will be
0300	0700–1200	1200–2200	1700–0800	initial
0400	1100–1800	1300–2200	1800–0800	starting
0500	1200	1400	1800–0800	time.
0600	1200	1400	1900–0800	
0700	1200	1400	2000	
0800	1300–1800	1500–2200	2000	
0900	1300–1800	1500–2200	2000	
1000	1700–2400	1600–2200	2100–0800	
1100	1800	2000–0600	2100–0800	
1200	1800	2100–0600	2200–0800	
1300	1800	2200	2200–0800	
1400	1900–2400	2200	2300–0800	
1500	1900–2400	2200	0500–2000	
1600	2300–0600	2300–0600	0600–2000	
1700	2400	2300–0600	0600–2000	
1800	2400	2400–0600	0700–2000	
1900	2400	0400–1400	0800	
2000	0100–0600	0500–1400	0800	
2100	0100–0600	0600	0800	
2200	0500–1200	0600	0900–2000	
2300	0600	0600	0900–2000	

- Hang first dose of antibiotic ASAP—don't wait to get on schedule. (You can potentially shorten the patient's length of stay depending on how quickly you hang the first dose.)
- Antibiotics ordered by pharmacokinetics (for example: gentamicin, vancomycin, etc.) are an exception to the above schedule. Pharmacy will inform you regarding the scheduling of these drugs.
- If a staggered time extends into the next day's MAR, make sure to indicate on the next day's MAR when the next dose is due.
- If you must deviate from the standard times, make sure to communicate this to Pharmacy, but BEWARE—any doses already dispensed by Pharmacy need to be corrected on the next day's MAR by the nurse doing that evening's MAR check.

GARDEN CITY HOSPITAL

Sliding-Scale Insulin Protocol for Adults

1. Check blood glucose with glucometer before meals and at bedtime if patient is eating or every 6 hours if the patient is not eating.
2. Administer regular human insulin subcutaneously according to the following dosage schedule:

Glucose Result	Coverage
<60 * STAT random blood sugar by lab draw. Call House Officer and notify of lab results.	
60–150	No coverage
151–200	5 units
201–250	10 units
251–300	15 units
301–350	20 units
351–400	25 units
> 400 STAT random blood sugar by lab draw. Give insulin; call House Officer with results. Recheck One Touch in 2 hours.	30 units

3. This protocol is optional for prescribers.
4. This protocol is not recommended for patients in ketoacidosis.
5. Patients with a hematocrit < 25% or > 60% or dialysis patients require a lab draw for glucose due to limitations of the One Touch. (Refer to Nursing Policy and Procedure Manual, Metabolic/Endocrine Section, page 1, number 4.)
   - See Nursing Policy and Procedure Manual, Metabolic/Endocrine Section, page 8, Hypoglycemia Treatment.

NOT A PERMANENT PART OF THE PATIENT'S CHART

LATROBE AREA HOSPITAL

Heparin Protocol Dosing Order Sheet

(Protocol is recommended for the treatment of patients with DVT, PE, A. Fib., Unstable Angina, and Acute MI who have not received thrombolytics during this admission.)

1. **Weigh patient and record:** _______________ kgs or _______________ lbs
   (Weights expressed in pounds must be converted to kilograms for subsequent calculations.)

2. **Initial Therapy:**
   Bolus:
   Protocol: 75 units/kg = _______________ Units IV over 2 to 3 minutes
   Alternative: _____ units/kg = _______________ Units IV over 2 to 3 minutes
   Round dose to nearest 500 units. Do not exceed 10,000 units bolus.

   Infusion:
   Protocol: 15 units/kg/hour = _______________ units/hour
   Alternative: _____ units/kg/hour = _______________ units/hour
   Round dose to the nearest 50 units.
   Standard concentration is 25,000 units/500mL D5W (50 units/mL).

3. **Laboratory Procedure:**
   A. Draw baseline aPTT and CBC now, if not already done within the past 24 hours.
   B. Initiate therapy and draw first aPTT in 6 hours.
   C. CBC with platelets every 3 days.
   D. Urinalysis and stool guaiac on initiation or within 24 hours.
   E. aPTT 6 hours after any dosage change, adjustment as per below sliding scale.
   *When 2 consecutive 6 hour aPTTs are therapeutic, order aPTT every AM while on heparin.

4. **Adjust heparin infusion according to sliding-scale below:**

Heparin Dosing Adjustment Instructions							
aPTT (sec)	Repeat Bolus (units)	Hold Infusion (hours)	Patients ≤ 200 lbs Adjust Rate (unit/hr)	Patients ≤ 200 lbs Adjust Rate (mL/hr)**	Patients > 200 lbs Adjust Rate (unit/hr)	Patients > 200 lbs Adjust Rate (mL/hr)**	Draw Next aPTT Test
<35	5000	0	↑ by 150	↑ by 3	↑ by 200	↑ by 4	6 hours
35–45	0	0	↑ by 100	↑ by 2	↑ by 150	↑ by 3	6 hours
46–70	0	0	0	0	0	0	Next AM*
71–80	0	0	↓ by 50	↓ by 1	↓ by 100	↓ by 2	6 hours
81–100	0	0.5	↓ by 100	↓ by 2	↓ by 150	↓ by 3	6 hours
>100	0	1.0	↓ by 150	↓ by 3	↓ by 200	↓ by 4	6 hours

** Valid infusion rate adjustments for standard dilution only (50 units/mL)

5. **Inspect** for abnormal bleeding or bruising, changes in mental status or level of consciousness, black tarry tools, hematuria, hemoptysis, or back pain every shift. If any of these occur, contact the physician immediately.

Physician Signature _______________ RN _______________ Date/Time _______________

White—Patient Chart Yellow—Pharmacy

METHODIST HOSPITAL/HEALTH SYSTEM MINNESOTA

Medication Administration Times for Food/Drug Interactions

Trade Name	Generic Name	Special Instructions	Time	Comments
ASA	aspirin	Take with food.	8:30 a.m.	Food helps to decrease GI irritation.
Capoten	captopril	Take on an empty stomach.	6—15—22	Food decreases absorption by 30–40% time as is tid or q8hr. 7–20 for BID schedule.
Carafate	sucralfate	Take on an empty stomach.	7:30—11:30—17—22	Sucralfate may bind to the protein in food.
Ceftin	cefuroxime	Take with whole milk or food; give HS snack with dose.	8:30—20:30	Milk increases absorption significantly (food less so).
Cipro	ciprofloxacin	Do not give with dairy products or Ca, Mg, or Fe supplements.	10—22	Ca, Mg, Fe can bind and inactivate Cipro.
Cortef	hydrocortisone	Take with food.	8:30—12:30—17:30—21	Food helps reduce GI irritation.
Cortone	cortisone	Take with food.	8:30 a.m.	Food helps reduce GI irritation.
Diabeta, Micronase	glyburide	Take 30 minutes before meals.	7:45—11:45—17	
Dilantin suspension	phenytoin suspension	Hold tube feedings 1 hour before and 2 hours after dose, give with or after meals.	8—14—20	Tube feedings may bind inactive phenytoin suspension.
Fosamax	alendronate	Take on an empty stomach—first thing in the morning: Give with a full glass of water. Patient should not lie down for about 1 hour after the dose.	6:30 a.m.	Calcium in food binds with the drug and inactivates it. Make sure to pull dose out of unit dose drawer before cart exchange.
Glucophage	metformin	Take with food.	8:30—17:30	Food decreases GI upset and helps increase compliance.
Glucotrol	glipizide	Take 30 minutes before meals.	7:45—11:45—17	
Indocin	indomethacin	Take with food.	8:30—12:30	Food helps reduce GI irritation.
Lanoxin	digoxin	Avoid high-fiber foods or products within 2 hours of dose.	11:00 a.m.	Fiber may reduce absorption or cause erratic absorption.
Lescol	fluvastatin	When ordered once a day, give in evening or HS.	22	Maximum cholesterol synthesis is at night.
Macrodantin, Macrobid	nitrofurantoin	Take with whole milk or food, give HS snack with dose.	8:30—12:30—17:30—21	Food significantly increases absorption.
Medrol	methyl-prednisolone	Take with food.	8:30—12:30—17:30—21	Food helps reduce GI irritation.

METHODIST HOSPITAL/HEALTH SYSTEM MINNESOTA

Medication Administration Times for Food/Drug Interactions (continued)

Trade Name	Generic Name	Special Instructions	Time	Comments
Motrin, Advil	ibuprofen	Take with food, give HS snack with dose.	8:30—12:30—17:30—21	Food helps reduce GI irritation.
multiple	potassium chloride	Take with food (do not hold now doses for empty stomach).	8:30—12:30—17:30—21	Food helps reduce GI irritation.
Naprosyn	naproxen	Take with food.	8:30—17:30	Food helps reduce GI irritation.
Orasone, Deltasone	prednisone	Take with food.	8:30 a.m.	Food helps reduce GI irritation.
Pepcid	famotidine	If ordered once a day, give HS.	22	Maximum output of stomach acid is at night.
Phoslo	calcium acetate	Take with meals.	8:30—12:30—17:30	Med works by binding phosphorous in food so it is not absorbed.
Pravachol	pravastatin	When ordered once a day, give in evening or at HS.	22	Maximum cholesterol synthesis is at night.
Precose	acarbose	Take with food.	8:30 a.m.	Food decreases GI upset and helps increase compliance. 8:15–9:45 acceptable.
Prilosec	omeprazole	Take before eating.	8:00+	Food decreases absorption. Give at 17:30 if BID.
Propulsid	cisapride	Take 1/2 hour AC (and if HS ordered).	7:30—11:30—17	Med stimulates gastric motility, so take before meals.
Relafen	nabumetone	Take with food.	8:30—17:30	Food helps reduce GI irritation.
Sumycin, others	tetracycline	Avoid foods high in Ca or Fe within 2 hours of dose.	6—11—16—22	Ca or Fe may bind and inactivate tetracycline. Time as is for qid or q6hr.
Tagamet	cimetidine	If ordered once a day, give HS.	22	Maximum output of stomach acid is at night.
Veetids, others	penicillin	Food decreases absorption, along with carbonated bev., and citrus juice.	6—11—16—22	
Zantac	ranitidine	If ordered once a day, give at bedtime (unless patient has symptoms during the day).	8:30—22	Gastric acid production increases at night.
Zithromax	azithromycin	Take on an empty stomach.	11:00 a.m.	Food decreases absorption by up to 50%.
Zocor	simvastatin	When ordered once a day, give in evening or HS.	22	Maximum cholesterol synthesis is at night.

Any HS dose on this list can be given earlier if the patient goes to bed early. Empty stomach is 2 hours after a meal and 1/2–1 hour before a meal. Meals on 5W are 8:15—12:15—17:30.

KAWEAH DELTA HEALTH CARE DISTRICT

Narcotic Flowsheet

Date ______________________________

Narcotic Ordered ______________________ Continuous Dose ______________________

PCA/Bolus Dose Frequency ____________ Titration Orders ______________________

Time	01	02	03	04	05	06	07	08	09	10	11	12	13	14	15	16	17	18	19	20	21	22	23	24
Sedation *(0–5) q 1h																								
Respirations q 1h																								
Initials																								
Document the following information every 4 hours and as needed																								
Pain intensity **(0–10)																								
Medication																								
Narcotic concentration (mg: cc)																								
Continuous rate (cc/hr)/dosage (mg)																								
PCA dosage (mg)																								
PCA/lock out (mins)																								
# Attempts																								
Loading dose																								
4 hour limit																								
Vial changed																								
Narcotic gtt Bolus (time and dose)																								
Total mg dispensed																								
q 4h																								
RN initials RN initials (verifying)																								

Signature ______________________

Signature ______________________

Signature ______________________

Signature ______________________

Signature ______________________

Signature ______________________

Signature ______________________

***Sedation Scale**

0 = Wide awake

1 = Drowsy

2 = Dozing intermittently

3 = Sleepy, responds to commands

4 = Responds only to tactile stimulation

5 = No response to tactile stimulation

**** Pain Intensity** 0 1 2 3 4 5 6 7 8 9 10

THUS FAR IN THE GUIDE, YOU HAVE LEARNED:

Part 1 *The Model for Improvement, which can be applied to any area you want to improve.*

Part 2 *A step-by-step guide to using that model to work on reducing adverse drug events, with each of the basic steps—setting aims, forming the team, establishing measures, and developing and testing changes—illustrated with examples.*

Part 3 *A group of change concepts that can be applied in different ways throughout the medication system to reduce adverse drug events.*

Part 4 *A comprehensive guide to reducing adverse drug events by improving the three major processes within the medication system: ordering, dispensing, and administration.*

Part 5

Troubleshooting: Overcoming Organizational Barriers

This section lists the most common barriers that organizations in the Breakthrough Series encountered in their efforts to reduce adverse drug events and describes the solutions that have proven most effective for each of those barriers.

Troubleshooting Overcoming Organizational Barriers

Setting Aims

BARRIER	SOLUTIONS
Multiple aims. Aims lack unity.	• Clarify aims. As long as the aims do not conflict, agree that the team will have a multiple focus; work toward unifying the aims as the project develops. If aims conflict, enlist the aid of the senior leader to obtain resolution.
Aim relates to only part of a system of care. Aim is not connected to the overall system.	• Starting with parts of a system is okay, but be ready to expand the scope of the project once initial aims are achieved.
Inability to agree on an aim. Aims focus only on individual parts of the process.	• Revisit the entire medication system and identify the parts that are most vulnerable to error (the critical control points), especially those that cross departmental boundaries. Focus the aim around these areas, rather than around any single department's turf. • Bring senior leadership into the discussion to align aims with the organization's strategic goals. • Refocus on the safe, accurate, and efficient delivery of medications to the patient. • Look for win-win arrangements. • Have people visit each other's departments or units to observe work directly.
Inability to select numerical goals	• Rather than seeking to reduce errors by a certain amount, specify parts of the system that could be made error free and set stretch goals around zero-defect performance.

See Part 4, Achieving Breakthrough Improvement in Reducing Adverse Drug Events, The Medication System.

Using Measurement

BARRIER	SOLUTIONS
Lack of clarity about how to define and measure the primary outcome measure (for example, reduction in adverse drug events)	• Use the aim as a reference for defining the outcome measure. Aims should specify numerical goals that reflect the change in the system. The team could define at the outset what it would like results to show at the end of the project and devise appropriate measures to track progress frequently over time.
Delays due to waiting for the information services department to provide data	• Use sampling and collect your own data instead of waiting for the information services department to produce the analysis. The team can compare the results from a small sample with those for a larger group at a later time. • Explore and use paper-and-pencil data collection while waiting for the information services department.
Limited access or no access to information services or to a computer system	• Use available resources and "just enough" data. Updating the organization's computer system is not feasible for a short-term project.
Resistance to small-scale data collection on the grounds of lack of scientific validity	• Differentiate between the level of data sophistication needed for research and that needed for improvement: randomized clinical trials are needed to *establish* standards of practice but not to test the best methods for putting existing knowledge into practice. • Use sampling to monitor the effects of small-scale tests of change. Once changes have been tested and implemented, collect additional data to verify results. Sampling is based on sound scientific principles and can satisfy many concerns about validity.

Using Measurement (continued)

BARRIER	SOLUTIONS
Not enough resources for data collection	• Make it easy for staff to collect data at the point of care by integrating data collection into their daily routine. For example, have a box in the pharmacy where pharmacists place a copy of each order they had to clarify. Or place a checksheet on the medication administration record (MAR) so that when the night nurses do reconciliations, they can check off the type of change. • Solicit the help of volunteers, students, or underutilized staff. • Reconsider how much data the team is collecting and establish sampling strategies that take less effort (for example, 2 hours per week instead of 4).
Measures don't show improvement after changes are made.	• Revisit what is being measured. Outcomes even for effective changes may take longer than a few months to emerge. • Continue to measure the outcome for the defined sample. Concurrently, check to ensure that the change is really taking place. (Are staff complying with guidelines? Are staff using the new communication system or transcription process?) • Document potential ADEs averted; for example, measure the number of doses of IV potassium given in dilute form.
Difficulty of measuring rare events (i.e., "We cannot reduce what we never had.")	• For infrequent events or hazards that have not been a problem, document potential ADEs averted. Examples include IV potassium given in dilute form and doses of benodiazepines within therapeutic range for people over 65.
Lack of reporting and fear of punishment	• Make sure staff understand that data will be used for learning and improvement, not for judgment and punishment. • Institute anonymous or confidential reporting of errors. • Grant immunity from punishment for reporting of errors. • Reward reporting of errors.
Managers resist anonymous reporting of errors or granting amnesty for reporting because they need leverage to discipline the "bad apples."	• Assist managers in finding other means of identifying incompetent staff. A truly incompetent nursing or medical staff member will evidence problems in addition to medication errors.

Team Functioning

BARRIER	SOLUTIONS
Ineffective teams	• Check team composition to make sure it includes day-to-day, system, and technical leadership. • Clarify the goals and keep the aim in focus. • Clarify roles, responsibilities, and time frames. • Define the goal and plan the overall strategy for achieving it. In addition to emphasizing "What can we do by next Tuesday?," focus on the ultimate goal of the project. Some teams pay so much attention to a particular series of tests of change that they lose sight of their overall goal. • Tap the energy and enthusiasm of many nurses, pharmacists, physicians, and others for improving the safety of the medication system.
Lack of representation from key disciplines	• Make sure that the team members represent the process the team is working to change. • Work with senior leadership to find a champion in the missing discipline and have the senior management arrange for his or her participation. • Raise the visibility of the improvement effort hospital-wide. Make it clear that this is not "a pharmacy project" or "a nursing project," but "a system project."
Lack of ownership of the process	• Establish owners for each part of the process. For example, the Chair of the Pharmacy and Therapeutics Committee owns drug choice and the formulary, the Pharmacy Director owns dispensing and disseminating information, the Vice President of Nursing or Patient Services owns administration and compliance with independent verification, and the Vice President for Medical Affairs owns the medication ordering process as it affects nurses, pharmacy, and patients. • Build these owners into an interdependent team. • Be sure to include "boundary spanners," people who work in both worlds, such as midlevel administrators, clinical pharmacists, and nursing and physician members of the Pharmacy and Therapeutics Committee.
Too large a team; difficulty meeting and scheduling	• Harness the interest and energy. Move some of the team members into work groups that can function simultaneously. • Ensure that the core improvement team meets weekly with no more than eight members, who together represent the key disciplines.

Team Functioning (continued)

BARRIER	SOLUTIONS
Lack of buy-in from physicians, nurses, or pharmacists	• Identify a physician or pharmacist champion. Choose a champion who is interested in reducing ordering errors and works with the Pharmacy and Therapeutics Committee. • Use the champion's improvements to convince others. • Instead of trying to build consensus among all of the physicians, work with those who want to work with the team on a test of change. • Identify pharmacists or key nursing personnel to work with physician champions. • Involve opinion leaders. Invite leaders from outside the local community to participate. • Secure administrative time for physicians, pharmacists, and nurses to work on the project. • Use a combination of strategies to secure physician buy-in, including providing feedback to providers, especially at the time of the order; using guidelines; and changing administrative policies to allow and encourage change.
Lack of time	• Plan productive team meetings. Establish rules for meetings and keep the team focused on the changes they are testing. • Take time at the beginning of each meeting to schedule the team's next meeting. • Use "huddles" between meetings. Some organizations find that they can accomplish a great deal in an informal "huddle" held for 5 minutes every day, or twice a week, in a hallway.

Developing and Testing Changes

BARRIER	SOLUTIONS
"We've tried to change things before, but nothing worked."	• Try to identify why previous efforts have failed. Separate out whether it was the idea for change or the attempt to implement it. • Emphasize that teams often learn more from failed tests than from successes. • Remember that the team will be testing small changes first, so there will be ample opportunity to identify and adjust to problems as they come up. • Emphasize the importance of studying the test to learn what really did happen. Many organizations abandon a change, assuming it "didn't work" because the outcome measure showed no evidence of change, when, in fact, the process was improved and in time would have shown excellent results.
Learning tests of change are often delayed for several weeks while waiting for tests to be completed.	• Avoid large-scale tests of change, which are often difficult to complete, absorbing time and energy. Tests should be short but significant. Test a big idea in a short time frame on a few subjects or in a limited location, so that the team can identify ways to modify and improve the change. • Always schedule time for reflection on tests.
Tests of change are not connected to the aim.	• In planning a test of change ("Plan") and reflecting on what was learned from the test ("Study"), make sure the change helps to achieve the aim. • Plot outcome measures related to the aim over time.
No one can identify changes that seem to apply to the project.	• Start by working on one of "The Basics" or any of the other changes suggested in the Guide (see Part 4, Achieving Breakthrough Improvement in Reducing Adverse Drug Events, The Basics). • Brainstorm with front line staff to identify the "errors waiting to happen" and what can be changed to prevent them. • Use the most powerful change concepts (for example, "Standardize," "Simplify") to generate ideas for improvement.

Developing and Testing Changes (continued)

BARRIER	SOLUTIONS
Resistance to testing	• Be sure that the team has a champion on the front line who is interested in shepherding the changes. Work with those who want to work with you. • Reassure staff that the team will be starting with very small tests (two patients, one afternoon, etc.) and watching closely to ensure that no new errors are being created. • Identify other concerns, such as "standardization is cookbook medicine," and address these concerns directly with information about how such standardization helps. • If clinicians resist multidisciplinary tests of change, start with some tests that nursing or pharmacy can implement alone and publicize the results widely.
Disagreement among team members about which changes to test first	• Use multivoting or other group process tools to make a quick decision about where to start. • Select changes that will yield quick results and improved processes for staff. • Reiterate that there will be lots of changes tested and that these are only the first. • Test more than one change at a time.
Lack of resources for testing and monitoring progress	• Use the internal quality improvement staff for facilitation or for collecting, analyzing, and reporting data. • Use the work of others described in this Guide. Teams also often get ideas from sharing with colleagues in other organizations, at professional meetings, and at conferences. Adapt and test ideas in the local setting. • Conduct quarterly "interest group" meetings for champions to share successes and provide continuing reinforcement. • Reframe the scope of the project if necessary. For example, test a change in only one department or only one clinic. • Make sure that the team leader is a subject matter expert or line manager, someone who is familiar with the day-to-day work.

Organizational Change Issues

BARRIER	SOLUTIONS
Lack of cooperation among departments	• Bring staff from other departments into the project. For example, invite staff from transport services and information services to participate on the team. • Focus on the common goal of safer patient care. • Seek the assistance of a senior leader who has an understanding of the system as a whole. • Thank those from outside the team who helped make the project work.
Impact of other change initiatives	• Align the project with the strategic goals of the organization. • Stress that this is a bottom-up approach. Other change initiatives may not have been effective because they were perceived as being imposed on the organization, whereas this project is driven by those who are actively involved in the process. • Utilize external requirements—for example, NCQA and JCAHO accreditation visits—to build support for change. • Build on initiatives that are currently under way in the same area whenever possible. (Sometimes, however, it is best to make a clean break, learn from past experience, and start fresh with a new approach.) • Explain the benefits of testing ideas on a small scale rather than waiting until a solution is fully developed.
Lack of senior leadership support	• Send reports of outcomes to the senior leader. • Invite the senior leader to a team meeting. • Share national media coverage with the senior leader.

Organizational Change Issues (continued)

BARRIER	SOLUTIONS
Lack of senior leadership support (continued)	**Tips for Senior Leaders:** The commitment of senior leadership is an important variable in an organization's ability to achieve breakthrough improvement. Senior leadership commitment doesn't have to be time-consuming in order to be strong and effective. The following are 10 simple but significant things senior leaders can do to create and sustain a culture of improvement: • Establish "stretch aims" or "stretch goals." Show by your constancy and commitment that you intend to do what is necessary in the organization to achieve a new level of performance. State and restate the aims. • Monitor the process frequently. To really accelerate improvement, review progress weekly or daily if necessary. • Stay in touch with the improvement effort. Support the team leader. Phone the leader. Pay specific, personal attention. • Visit the team. Drop in on meetings, if only for a few minutes. • Visit the site of the change. For example, visit the pharmacy or the intensive care unit; show that you are aware of the improvement work being done. Look at the charts that monitor progress. Ask how you, as an executive, can be more helpful. • Move the review of the progress of the improvement effort up on the agenda. Make it clear that improvement has high priority in the organization.

Organizational Change Issues (continued)

BARRIER	SOLUTIONS
Lack of senior leadership support (continued)	• Make sure that the team has the resources it needs. For example, the team may need designated staff time or access to key data that others have collected. • Celebrate successes. Public celebrations of improvement efforts or personal expressions of appreciation are just as important as any modification of pay structure. • Keep the bigger system in view. The many local improvements are connected in a larger way to the system as a whole. It is the job of senior leaders to keep sight of, and help others to see, this larger context. • Encourage team members to visit or work with other organizations, including travel to other locations. It may be one of the senior leader's wisest investments.

In this section, you will find a variety of resources to help you reduce adverse drug events in your organization:

Part 6

Resources for Reducing Adverse Drug Events

Breakthrough Series Assessment

The Planning Group developed the following assessment tool to determine to what extent the Breakthrough Series Collaborative on Reducing Adverse Drug Events met its stated goals. Organizations engaged in making changes to achieve breakthrough improvement may find this tool useful in assessing their own progress.

The Breakthrough Series is built on the belief that organizations working together for 10 to 12 months, learning the latest scientific information available on improving a specific area of health care, and finding practical and effective means to put that knowledge into practice, can achieve breakthrough results.

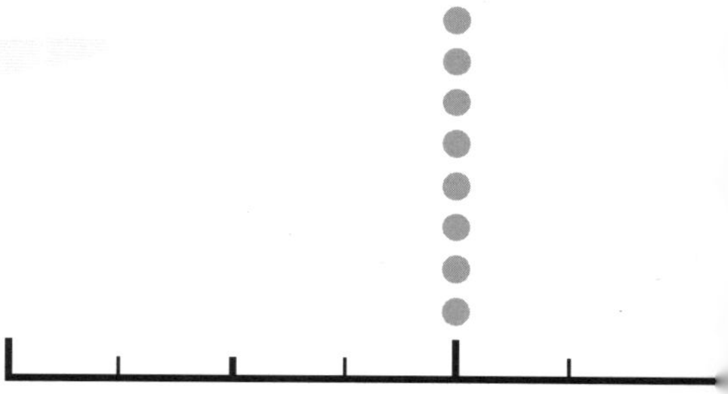

1

Nonstarter

The organization attended the first Learning Session of the Collaborative but did not initiate any improvement activity.

2

Activity but no changes

The organization actively engaged in the effort, but its initiatives did not include any changes in practice. For example, the team conducted a literature search or collected data, but did not make changes.

Organizations in the Collaborative on Reducing Adverse Drug Events worked on many different aspects of the total system of medication ordering, dispensing, and administration, and set stretch goals for their work over the 12-month period.

The specific goal of the Collaborative on Reducing Adverse Drug Events was clear and ambitious: Reduce adverse drug events by 30% or more within 12 months. An assessment of 4 on the scale in Figure 6.1 would be consistent with that goal.

THE ASSESSMENT SCALE RATES ORGANIZATIONS ACCORDING TO FIVE CATEGORIES:

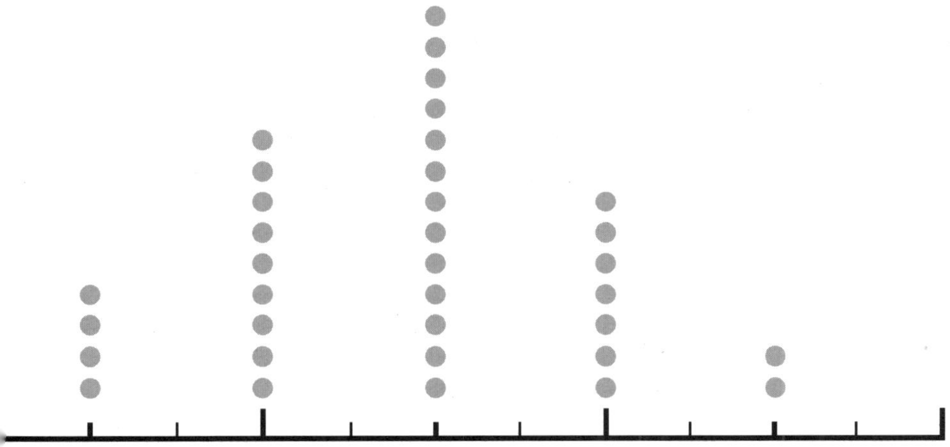

Figure 6.1
Assessment: Breakthrough Series Collaborative on Reducing Adverse Drug Events (March 1996–March 1997)

The assessment is a consensus of the Planning Group and the Collaborative organizations.

3
Modest improvement

- The team collected anecdotal evidence about changes.
- Data-related evidence showed improvement (10% to 30% of the stated goal) in a localized process—for example, a 20% reduction in late medications on 5 West.
- A large system showed early indications of improvement—for example, a 20% reduction in nonstandard orders in the pharmacy.

4
Significant progress

- A significant improvement (100% of the stated goal) occurred at the level of a major subsystem—for example, a 30% reduction in serious errors in the ICU.
- A significant improvement (100% of the stated goal) occurred at the system level for a cohort of patients—for example, a 50% reduction in incorrect doses for elderly patients.

5
Outstanding, sustainable results

- An outstanding improvement (100% of the stated goal) occurred at the system level—for example, a 50% reduction in serious errors (preventable ADEs) for all patients.
- The organization achieved levels at the leading edge—for example, error reduction rates were greater than those specified in the Collaborative goals.

Key Contacts

Collaborative Chair

Lucian L. Leape, MD
Adjunct Professor of Health Policy
Department of Health Policy
and Management
Harvard School of Public Health
Boston, MA

Collaborative Director

Andrea Kabcenell, RN, MPH
Institute for Healthcare Improvement
Boston, MA

Baptist Medical Center, Columbia

Taylor at Marion Street
Columbia, SC 29220

Karen Baxley
Clinical Nurse Specialist
Tel: (803) 771-5892
Fax: (803) 988-8520
E-mail: KOBAXLEY@bhsc.hbocvan.com

Beth Israel Deaconess Medical Center

One Deaconess Road
Boston, MA 02215

Nancy Wilkinson, RN
Senior Staff Consultant
Tel: (617) 632-8269
Fax: (617) 632-7887
E-mail: nwilkins@nedhmail.nedh.harvard.edu

Blue Cross and Blue Shield of Massachusetts

100 Summer Street
Mail Stop 01/07
Boston, MA 02110-2190

Paula Griswold
Director, Health Institution Performance
Partnership
Tel: (617) 832-3639

The Cambridge Hospital

1493 Cambridge Street
Cambridge, MA 02139-1099

Dodi Huang-Hellinger, RPh
Pharmacy Supervisor/Co-Chair Nursing
Tel: (617) 498-1324
Fax: (617) 498-2228

Cedars-Sinai Medical Center
8700 Beverly Boulevard
Los Angeles, CA 90043

Frank Saya, PharmD
Assistant Director, Pharmacy Services
Tel: (310) 855-5611
Fax: (310) 854-4937
E-mail: Saya@CSMC.edu

Children's Hospital, Boston
300 Longwood Avenue
Boston, MA 02115

Frank Federico, RPh
Director of Pharmacy
Tel: (617) 355-6847
Fax: (617) 731-5471
E-mail: federico@a1.tch.harvard.edu

Children's Hospital of Philadelphia
34th Street and Civic Center Blvd.
Nursing Administration
Philadelphia, PA 19104

Jane Barnsteiner, PhD, RN
Director, Nursing Practice and Research
Tel: (215) 590-3147
Fax: (215) 590-4439
Email: barnsteiner@email.chop.edu

Dana-Farber Cancer Institute
44 Binney Street
The Dana Building, Room 1530
Boston, MA 02115

Silvia Bartel, RPh
Director of Pharmacy
Tel: (617) 632-2110
Fax: (617) 632-2254
E-mail: sylvia_bartel@dfci.harvard.edu

Dartmouth-Hitchcock Medical Center
One Medical Center Drive
Lebanon, NH 03756

Jean T. Avery, RN
Clinical Quality Associate
Tel: (603) 650-8280
Fax: (603) 650-4900
E-mail: Jean.Avery@Hitchcock.org

Deaconess-Nashoba Hospital
200 Groton Road
Ayer, MA 01432

Gail Kerwood, RN, MEd
Vice President for Patient Care Services
Tel: (508) 722-0200 ext 210
Fax: (508) 772-8112
E-mail: gkerwood@nedhmail.nedh.harvard.edu

Deaconess-Waltham Hospital
Hope Avenue
Waltham, MA 02154

Madeline O'Reilly, RN
Director, Pharmacy Services
Tel: (617) 647-6690
Fax: (617) 647-6007

Fairview Health System
6401 France Avenue South
Minneapolis, MN 55435

Steven Meisel, PharmD
Assistant Director, Pharmacy
Tel: (612) 924-5894
Fax: (612) 924-1511
E-mail: smeisel1@fairview.org

Kaiser Foundation Health Plan, Inc.
Department of Quality
One Kaiser Plaza
Oakland, CA 94612

Sharon Conrow
Vice President, Quality
Tel: (510) 271-5956
Fax: (510) 271-6836

- **Kaiser Permanente, Northern California Region**
  1950 Franklin Street
  Oakland, CA 94612

  Nancy Carlson, RN
  Assistant Leader, Regional Patient Care Services
  Tel: (510) 987-4001
  Fax: (510) 873-5288
  E-Mail: REHNEC@ncal.kaiperm.org

- **Kaiser Permanente, Southern California Region**
  410 North Lakeview Ave.
  Anaheim, CA 92807

  Carey C. Cotterell, RPh
  Area Chief Pharmacist, Orange County
  Tel: (714) 279-4706
  Fax: (714) 279-4689
  E-mail: carey.c.cotterell@kp.org

Kaweah Delta Health Care District
400 West Mineral King
Visalia, CA 93291

Susan Bates, RN
Renal Team Coordinator
Tel: (209) 625-7202
Fax: (209)635-4026
E-mail: sbates@kdhcd.org

Kimball Medical Center
600 River Avenue
Lakewood, NJ 08701

Patricia A. Cook, RPh
Director of Pharmaceutical Services
Tel: (732) 363-1900 ext 2832
Fax: (732) 886-4679

Jeanette Wilson, RN
Performance Improvement/Standards Coordinator
Tel: (732) 363-1900 ext 2301
Fax: (732) 886-4679

Loss Prevention Foundation
50 North Perry Street
Pontiac, MI 48342

- **Bay Medical Center**
  1900 Columbus Avenue
  Bay City, MI 49708

  Ellen Talbott, RN
  Director of Nursing
  Tel: (517) 894-8610
  Fax: (517) 894-6114
  E-mail: ET2404@AOL.com

- **Garden City Hospital**
  6245 Inkster Road
  Garden City, MI 48135

  Lisa Cayo
  Clinical Coordinator, Pharmacy
  Tel: (313) 485-4465
  Fax: (313) 421-3530
  E-mail: lisacayo@l.imap.itd.umich.edu

- **Mt. Clemens General Hospital**
  1000 Harrington Boulevard
  Mt. Clemens, MI 48043

  Lee Holmberg, MA, CP, HQ
  Administrative Director
  Quality and Resource Management
  Tel: (810) 493-8094
  Fax: (810) 493-8717
  E-mail: lholmberg@mcgh.org

- **Pontiac Osteopathic Hospital Medical Center**
  50 North Perry Street
  Pontiac, MI 48342

  Lawrence Abramson, DO, MPH
  Quality Assessment Director
  Tel: (248) 338-5510
  Fax: (248) 338-5667
  E-mail: ljabramson@aol.com

Lucile Salter Packard Children's Hospital at Stanford
725 Welch Road
Palo Alto, CA 94304

Nancy Carragee, RN, MS
Director, Quality Management
Tel: (415) 497-8096
Fax: (415) 497-8465
E-mail: rn.npc@lpch.stanford.edu

Maine Medical Center
22 Bramhall Street
Portland, ME 04102

Paul M. Cox, Jr., MD
Associate Vice President for Medical Quality
Tel: (207) 871-2018
Fax: (207) 871-4610
E-mail: coxp@mail.mmc.org

Mercy Hospital
3663 South Miami Avenue
Miami, FL 33133

Michael J. Clark, PharmD
Director of Pharmacy
Tel: (305) 285-2632
Fax: (305) 285-2903
E-mail: gatorx@ix.netcom.com

Methodist Hospital/HealthSystem Minnesota
6500 Excelsior Boulevard
St. Louis Park, MN 55426

Ronald Kitzmann
Director of Pharmacy, HealthSystem Minnesota
Tel: (612) 993-5445
Fax: (612) 993-6813
E-mail: 36178@hsm1.hsmnet.com

Morton Plant Mease Health Care
601 Main Street
Dunedin, FL 34698

J. Mike Bishop, RPh, MS
Director of Pharmaceutical Services
Tel: (813) 734-6816
Fax: (813) 734-6405

Munson Medical Center
1105 Sixth Street
Traverse City, MI 49684

Terry Hasslinger
Continuous Quality Improvement Administrator
Tel: (616) 935-6536
Fax: (616) 935-7174
E-mail: nicholl4@pilot.msu.edu

North Iowa Mercy Health Center
1000 4th Street SW
Mason City, IA 50401

Mike Ahrens, RPh
Clinical Coordinator
Pharmaceutical Services
Tel: (515) 422-7542
Fax: (515) 422-7431

Northwest Covenant Medical Center
25 Pocono Road
Denville, NJ 07670

Jesse Hagmeyer
Pharmacy Manager, Clinical Services
Tel: (201) 625-6002
Fax: (201) 625-6198

Paoli Memorial Hospital
255 West Lancaster Avenue
Paoli, PA 19301

Karen Taylor
Assistant Director, Record and Review Services
Tel: (610) 648-1425
Fax: (610) 296-2520

Promina Gwinnett Health System
PO Box 348
Lawrenceville, GA 30046

Marty Beaver, RN, CPHQ
Director, Nursing Clinical Education and Quality
Tel: (770) 995-4275
Fax: (770) 682-2249
E-mail: mbeaver123@aol.com

SSM Health Care
477 North Lindbergh Boulevard
St. Louis, MO 63141

Barbara A. Spreadbury
Corporate Director, Quality Resource Center
Tel: (314) 994-7747
Fax: (314) 994-7900
E-mail: bspreadbury@ssmhc.com

- **Good Samaritan Regional Health Center**
  605 North 12th Street
  Mount Vernon, IL 62864

  Jeralee Sargent
  Infection Control/Risk Management Coordinator
  Tel: (618) 241-2259
  Fax: (618) 241-5805

- **St. Marys Hospital Medical Center**
  707 South Mills Street
  Madison, WI 53715-0450

  Sherry Anderson, RN
  Nursing QI Coordinator
  Tel: (608) 258-6741
  Fax: (608) 259-5327
  E-mail: shanderson@ssmhc.com

Suburban Hospital
8600 Old Georgetown Road
Bethesda, MD 20814

William F. Minogue, MD
Senior Vice President for Medical Affairs
Tel: (310) 896-2579
Fax: (301) 897-1330
E-mail: wminoguemd@aol.com

United Hospital/Allina Health System
333 North Smith Avenue
St. Paul, MN 55102

Bruce Scott, MS
Director of Pharmacy
Tel: (612) 220-8844
Fax: (612) 220-5323

University of Chicago Hospitals and Health Systems
5841 S. Maryland Avenue, MC 0010
Chicago, IL 60637

Jeannell Mansur, PharmD
Director of Pharmaceutical Services
Tel: (773) 702-6242
Fax: (773) 702-6631
E-mail: jmansur@mcis.bsd.uchicago.edu

The Valley Hospital
223 North Van Dien Avenue
Ridgewood, NJ 07450

Michael Mutter
Assistant Director, Pharmacy
Tel: (201) 447-8121
Fax: (201) 447-8435
E-mail: mikemutter@aol.com

VHA East/New Jersey
Cranbury, NJ

- **Elizabeth General Medical Center**
  925 East Jersey Street
  Elizabeth, NJ 07201

  Barbara Butler, RN
  Director, Nursing Service
  Tel: (908) 629-8172
  Fax: (908) 629-8972

- **Grand View Hospital**
  700 Lawn Avenue
  Sellersville, PA 18960

  Carolyn Beck, RN, BS
  Quality Management Supervisor
  Tel: (215) 453-4212
  Fax: (215) 453-4341

- **Lehigh Valley Hospital**
  1200 South Cedar Crest Boulevard
  PO Box 689
  Allentown, PA 18105-1556

  Fred Pane
  Director, Pharmacy
  Tel: (610) 402-8881
  Fax: (610) 402-8817
  E-mail: fred.pane@lvh.com

VHA Pennsylvania
415 Holiday Drive
Pittsburgh, PA 15220

Marjorie Devett
Consultant, Clinical Improvement
Tel: (412) 922-9124
Fax: (412) 922-1672
E-mail: mdevett@vha.com

- **Allegheny General Hospital**
  320 East North Avenue
  Pittsburgh, PA 15212

  Marge Hardt
  Senior Director, Nursing
  Tel: (412) 359-8198
  Fax: (412) 359-3678
  E-mail: hardt@pgh.auhs.edu

- **Latrobe Area Hospital**
  121 West Second Avenue
  Latrobe, PA 15650-1096

  Dean Matanin, PharmD
  Director of Pharmacy
  Tel: (412) 537-1249
  Fax: (412) 537-1265

Wesley Medical Center
550 North Hillside, Suite 104
Wichita, KS 67214

Bob Ragan, RPh, MHS
Pharmacy Manager
Tel: (316) 688-3379
Fax: (316) 688-7093
E-mail: 73170.1222@compuserve.com

Quality Improvement Storyboards

Storyboards are a valued tool of the Breakthrough Series for effectively presenting an organization's work to a variety of audiences—to other organizations within each Collaborative, to the larger audience at each National Congress, and to the home audience within each organization.

In preparing storyboards, organizations in the Breakthrough Series use the following guidelines.

PURPOSE

A storyboard is a presentation of a project in a poster fashion for others to examine. Its purpose is to communicate a story—the story of the work that has been performed.

GOAL

The goal of a storyboard presentation is to capture the reader's attention quickly and to communicate the desired information clearly and succinctly.

Key Characteristics

Creativity should play a part in storyboard design, but teams should design the presentation so that it can be understood in a brief period of time. Complex charts or tables diminish viewers' ability to comprehend the content rapidly, and designers should avoid them. Likewise, presenting too much information overwhelms viewers and diminishes the impact of the presentation.

- Design for ease of comprehension and readability.
- Include only critical information.
- Keep it simple.
- Tell the truth without fudging.
- Make the goal of the project readily apparent.
- Describe interventions concisely.
- Display data over time in a run chart, annotating what changes were made, when.
- Outline conclusions based on the data.
- Present plans for implementation or further testing of changes.

Storyboard Outline

1. **Organization name and location**
   (city and state)

2. **Aim**
   State the aim succinctly, including a numerical goal and a time frame for achieving it.

3. **Measures**
   - Define one to three key outcome measures.
   - Describe the sampling plan: What data will be collected, when?
   - Include an annotated time series graph of the key outcome measures.
   - Clearly label the X- and Y-axes.
   - Indicate the sample size.
   - Indicate on the graphs when changes were tested.

4. **Changes**
   Briefly describe each of the changes indicated on the graphs.

5. **Results**
   State the results achieved to date: What numerical goals were achieved, in what amount of time?

SAMPLE STORYBOARDS

St. Marys Hospital Medical Center
Madison, WI

Aim

Standardize IV antibiotic schedules:

- Prevent delay in therapy by standardizing the dosing schedule between Nursing and Pharmacy.
- Start the second dose within the standard time.
- Start the first dose ASAP (within 2 hours of Unit Clerk's transcription).
- Start the first dose within 2 hours of admission.

Background

- Guidelines to initiate therapy and reach standard administration times did not exist.
- Practice variation resulted in the following:
  38% of antibiotics took more than 2 hours to start therapy.
  38% of antibiotics were not administered within standard dosing schedules.

Measures

- Percentage of standard times utilized

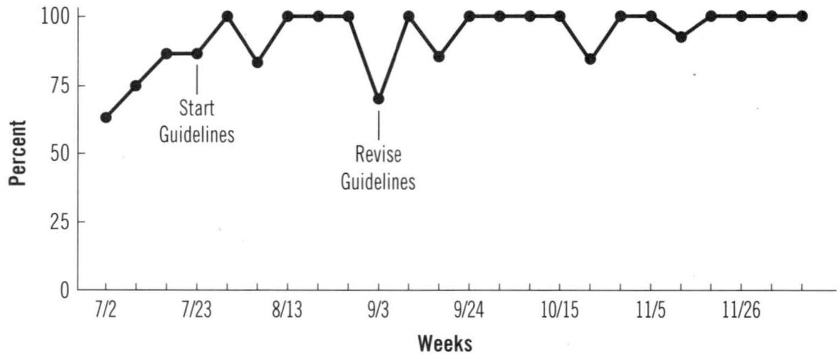

- Percentage of first doses administered within 2 hours of Unit Clerk's transcription

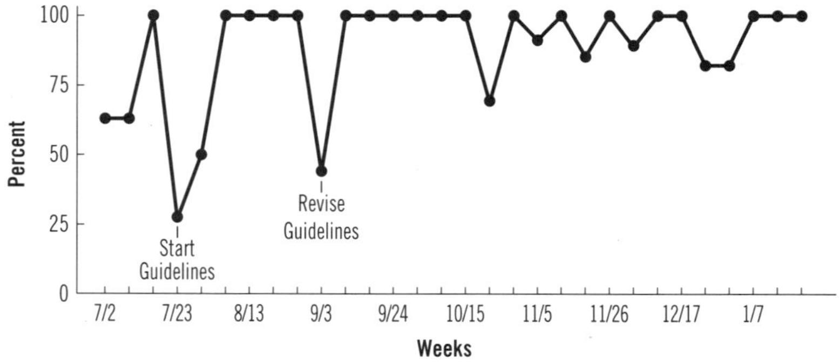

St. Marys Hospital Medical Center
Madison, WI (continued)

- Percentage of first doses administered within 2 hours of admission

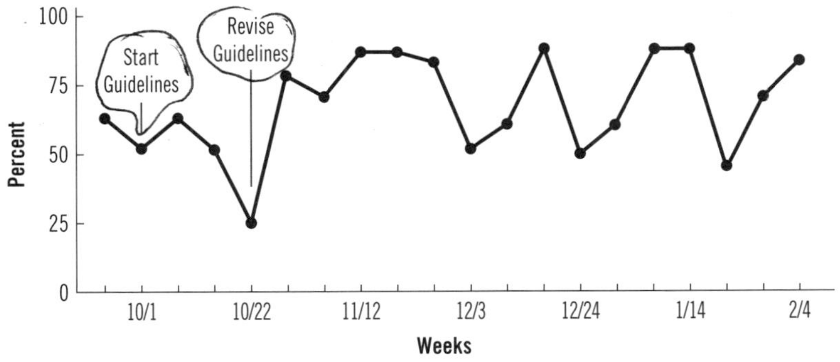

Changes

1. Develop and pilot an anonymous Incident Report "Short Form" including "near misses."
2. Standardize the times antibiotics are given without delaying therapy.
   - Develop a scheduling tool to determine when the next dose is due.
   - Implement the scheduling tool on a pilot unit.
   - Clarify and revise the scheduling tool.
   - Implement the scheduling tool throughout the hospital.
3. Administer the first dose of IV antibiotics ASAP (within 2 hours of Unit Clerk's review).
   - Define and implement the standard on a pilot unit.
   - Implement the standard throughout the hospital.
   - Change the standard to be within 2 hours of admission.

Results

An easy-to-use reference table that standardizes the dosing schedule between nursing and pharmacy has significantly decreased the delay in patient therapy and omissions relating to IV antibiotics. The team achieved the following goals:

- The percentage of antibiotic doses given at standard times increased from a mean of 60% to a mean of 98%.
- The percentage of antibiotic doses given within 2 hours of admission increased from a mean of 50% to a mean of 70%.
- The percentage of first-dose antibiotics given within 20 minutes of Unit Clerk's transcription increased from a mean of 60% to a mean of 92%.

Improvement Cycle Worksheet

Organizations in the Breakthrough Series use the following format to document and report their work on testing changes. Each Improvement Cycle Worksheet documents one Plan-Do-Study-Act (PDSA) cycle.

BREAKTHROUGH SERIES COLLABORATIVE ON REDUCING ADVERSE DRUG EVENTS

IMPROVEMENT CYCLE WORKSHEET

Organization: Pontiac Osteopathic Hospital Medical Center
Team Leader: Dr. Abramson
Cycle Number: 2: Reduce distractions
Began: 8/27/96
Completed: 9/30/96

Overall Aim: Reduce adverse drug events on the cardiac monitoring unit (CMU) by 50% within 12 months.

Objective of This Cycle: Reduce distractions associated with the unit dose cart exchange process.

PLAN

Describe the plans for the cycle: who, what, where, when, and how data will be collected.

Who: Pharmacy
What: Change work day for pharmacy
Where: Pharmacy, all nursing units
When: Effective 9/29/96

How:
Change 1: Proposed new work day:

0200 Nurses complete medication administration record (MAR) reconciliation forms and send to pharmacy for corrections.
0530 RPh generates unit dose fill lists for cart fill.
0600 Two day shift technicians report to work and start unit dose cart fill process.
0700 Day shift RPh reports to work and begins cart check process along with night shift RPh.
0800 Checked unit dose carts are delivered to patient-specific rooms in locked cabinets. Yesterday's drawer is removed and returned to pharmacy.
0900 Cart exchange completed. Med crediting begins and is completed before end of afternoon shift.
1000 Floor stock requests from nursing units are completed and forwarded to pharmacy.
1430 Deadline for floor stock to be resupplied to nursing units.
2100 MAR and IV fluid records generated for the next day.
2200 MAR and IV fluid records delivered to floors for nurse reconciliation.

Change 2: Technician shifts will be changed to 0600–1430.

Change 3: Increase floor stock of IVs. All large volumes except those containing additives will be on the nursing unit.

IMPROVEMENT CYCLE WORKSHEET (continued)

Measures to be used:

- Incidence rate of missing medication (a major distraction for nursing and pharmacy) Pharmacy will collect data hospital-wide. Data collection will begin immediately for baseline determination prior to implementation of the new process. Pharmacy will collect missing med label sheets, measure total missing doses/total doses dispensed. Four weeks after implementation, pharmacy will attempt to obtain reason for missing med and identify trends.

DO

What actually happened when we tested the changes? What did we observe?

The nurses immediately reported that the new unit dose cart exchange time significantly improved their processes and reduced distractions associated with the prior 1400 delivery time. No problems were encountered with technician time shifts. The pharmacy technicians also reported fewer distractions during the cart fill time in the early morning as opposed to the prior midmorning work period. The pharmacists noted fewer corrections prior to release of the carts.

STUDY

What were the results? (Include data and narrative.) What do we conclude?

The incidence rate from baseline to 3 days after implementation shows initial reduction in missing doses. Prior to the change, the average daily missing dose incidence was 0.0085 compared to the post-change rate of 0.0049.

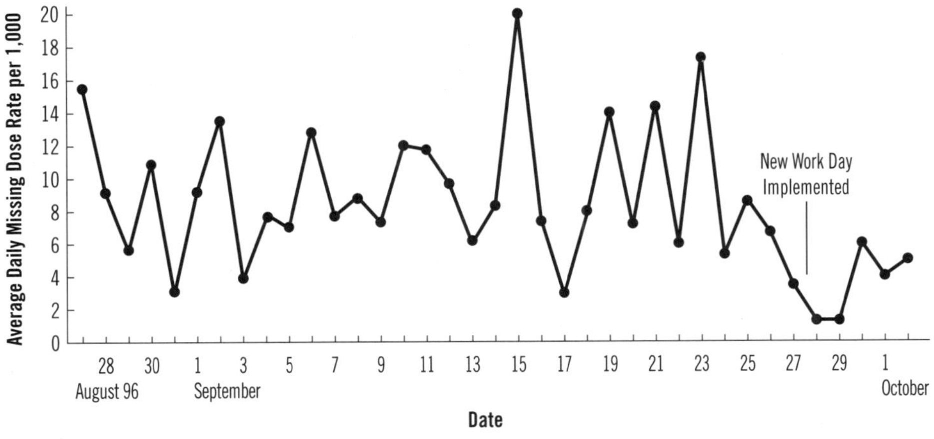

ACT

What are the objectives of the next cycle?

- Continue process.
- Follow up at 4 weeks.
- Address distractions associated with late or missing IVPB medications by delivering them earlier.

Annotated Bibliography

GENERAL LITERATURE ON QUALITY IMPROVEMENT

Berwick D. Continuous improvement as an ideal in health care. *N Engl J Med.* 1989;320:53-56.

A classic, one of the first published calls for systems thinking in clinical care.

Berwick DM, Godfrey AB, Roessner J. *Curing Health Care: New Strategies for Quality Improvement.* San Francisco, CA: Jossey-Bass Publishers; 1990.

This book explains how health care leaders can apply methods of modern quality management in their organizations to improve efficiency and safety, achieve new breakthroughs in performance, reduce costs, and help reshape our troubled health care system. Drawing on the experiences and lessons of the National Demonstration Project on Quality Improvement in Health Care, the authors show how quality management techniques adopted from industry can be applied to solve specific problems in health care.

Eye on Improvement. Boston, MA: Institute for Healthcare Improvement.

This newsletter, which publishes abstracts of articles from about 50 different journals in 24 yearly issues, provides an effective way to keep up with the rapidly expanding amount of literature devoted to continuous quality improvement. (Editorial office: PO Box 2730, Chino Valley, AZ 86323; (800) 895-4951.)

Gaucher EJ, Coffey RJ. *Total Quality in Health Care: From Theory to Practice.* San Francisco, CA: Jossey-Bass Publishers; 1993.

As the title suggests, the authors link theory to practice in continuous quality improvement, based on their experience implementing quality management at the University of Michigan Medical Center. Chapter 7 explores the role of physicians.

Goldfield N, Nash DB, eds. *Providing Quality Care: The Challenge to Clinicians.* 2nd ed. Philadelphia, PA: American College of Physicians; 1995.

Provides a summary of the work of leading researchers in health services research, with an editorial commentary at the end of each chapter.

Langley G, Nolan K, Nolan T, Norman C, Provost L. *The Improvement Guide: A Practical Approach to Enhancing Organizational Performance.* San Francisco, CA: Jossey-Bass Publishers; 1996.

This book provides critical information about improvement and formed the basis for many ideas in this Guide.

Nolan T, Schall M. *Reducing Delays and Waiting Times Throughout the Healthcare System*. Boston, MA: Institute for Healthcare Improvement; 1996.
The first in a series of Breakthrough Series Guides designed to help organizations make major, rapid improvements. The Guide is based on the work of 27 health care organizations that worked together for a year to reduce delays and waiting times in surgery, the emergency department, and clinics and physicians' offices, and to increase access to care.

Plsek, PE. *Creativity, Innovation, and Quality*. Milwaukee, WI: ASQ Quality Press; 1997.
This book guides the reader through directed creativity from first principles to application. The first third of the book covers the theory of directed creativity, including the mechanics of the mind and heuristics for directed creativity. The second third presents the three principles behind all tools for creative thinking and reviews the hundreds of tools available. The final third covers the application of directed creativity to reengineering, design, customer needs analysis, and problem solving.

Weiss K, Mendoza G, Schall M, Berwick D, Roessner J. *Improving Asthma Care in Children and Adults*. Boston, MA: Institute for Healthcare Improvement; 1997.
The second in a series of Breakthrough Series Guides designed to help organizations make major, rapid improvements. The Guide is based on the work of 12 health care organizations that worked together for a year to improve asthma care in children and adults.

REDUCING ADVERSE DRUG EVENTS RECOMMENDED READING

Avorn J. Putting adverse drug events into perspective. *JAMA* 1997;277:341-342.
Editorial accompanying cost papers by Bates and Classen (below). Calls for a systems approach, citing these papers as evidence of its value. Avorn gives a well-deserved compliment to the often overlooked pharmacists and their role in heading off disasters. Notes that computers are powerful tools to deal with these problems.

Bates DW, Boyle DL, Vander Vliet MB, Schneider J, Leape LL. Relationship between medication errors and adverse drug events. *J Gen Int Med* 1995;10:199-205.
Results of a detailed study of the incidence of medication errors and their relationship to preventable adverse drug events.

Bates DW, Cullen DJ, Laird N, et al. Incidence of adverse drug events and potential adverse drug events: Implications for prevention. *JAMA* 1995;274:29-34.

A comprehensive and rigorous attempt to measure the extent of adverse drug events and one of the first studies to demonstrate that errors are common in the prescribing stage of the medication system. Events were discovered by stimulated voluntary reporting and daily reviews of the medical records. Because the study reported a much higher incidence of errors than previous reports, it has become a benchmark for the incidence of adverse drug events. (An ADE was found in 6.5% of admissions; 28% were due to errors and thus preventable.)

Bates DW, O'Neil AC, Boyle D, Teich J, et al. Potential identifiability and preventability of adverse events using information systems. *J Am Med Informatics Assoc* 1994; 1:404-411.

Description of the use of a computerized screening system that identifies potential adverse drug events by use of a logic system based on laboratory data and orders. Shows what can be done if all clinical and laboratory information is on-line.

Bates DW, Spell N, Cullen DJ, et al. The costs of adverse drug events in hospitalized patients. *JAMA* 1997;277:307-311.

Analysis of the costs of adverse drug events identified in Adverse Drug Event Prevention Study (see Bates et al., *JAMA* 1995 above), using a case-control methodology. Preventable adverse drug events cost twice as much as nonpreventable ADEs and averaged $4,685 each at one teaching hospital. Authors estimate that hospitals in the study are losing $2.8 million each year on preventable ADEs.

Bedell SE, Deitz DC, Leeman D, Delbanco TL. Incidence and characteristics of preventable iatrogenic cardiac arrests. *JAMA* 1991;265:2815-2820.

Landmark study that demonstrates that most cardiac arrests that occur in hospitals are caused by misuse of drugs and are, therefore, potentially preventable.

Brennan TA, Leape LL, Laird N, Hebert L, Localio AR, Lawthers AG, et al. Incidence of adverse events and negligence in hospitalized patients: Results of the Harvard Medical Practice Study I. *N Engl J Med* 1991;324:370-376.

Description of findings that nearly 4% of patients hospitalized in acute care hospitals suffer an injury caused by treatment.

Bogner MS, ed. *Human Error in Medicine*. Hillsdale, NJ: Lawrence Erlbaum; 1994.

This collection of (expanded) presentations from an AAAS symposium on error in medicine provides a good overview of many aspects of health care errors. A number of the key contributors to current thought concerning error in medicine are represented.

Christensen JF, Levinson W, Dunn PM. The heart of darkness: The impact of perceived mistakes on physicians. *J Gen Intern Med* 1992;7:424-31.

Gripping account of the effect of errors on physicians and their inability to deal with them or receive support when needed.

Classen DC, Pestotnik SL, Evans RS, Burke JP. Computerized surveillance of adverse drug events in hospital patients. *JAMA* 1991;266:2847-51.

Description of the continuous monitoring system at LDS Hospital in Salt Lake City, Utah. This is an impressive system that integrates clinical, laboratory, drug, and cost information to identify ADEs both prospectively and retrospectively.

Classen DC, Pestotnik SL, Evans RS, et al. Adverse drug events in hospitalized patients: Excess length of stay, extra costs, and attributable mortality. *JAMA* 1997;277:301-306.

Cost study from the LDS Salt Lake City group.

Cullen DJ, Bates DW, Small SD, et al. The incident reporting system does not detect adverse drug events: A problem in quality assurance. *Jt Com J Qual Improv* 1995;21:541-548.

A critical analysis of the incident reporting system. Makes the case that reliance on incident reports results in a drastic underestimate of the rates of events. The yield of spontaneous reporting of ADEs by the hospital incident reporting system was compared to intensive, confidential data collection by means of stimulated self-report and daily record review. Ninety-four percent of ADEs discovered by record review and confidential report were not reported as incident reports.

Kahneman D, Slovic P, Tversky A, eds. *Judgment Under Uncertainty: Heuristics and Biases*. New York, NY: Cambridge University Press; 1982.

The classic collection of studies of how humans make judgments under (usual) conditions of uncertainty. The authors coined some of the key terms in behavioral science.

Leape LL. Error in medicine. *JAMA* 1994;272:1851-1857.

An overview of the problems of detection and management of errors in health care. It explores the effects of errors on those who make them and reviews the cognitive basis for human error. The concept of systems failures as the cause of errors is introduced, and suggestions are made as to how hospitals can use human factors principles to redesign their systems for safety. For those new to the subject of error prevention, this is the best place to start.

Leape LL, Bates DW, Cullen DJ, et al. Systems analysis of adverse drug events. *JAMA* 1995;274:35-43.

The companion paper to the Bates study above, this report provides the results of the investigation of the causes of errors in the same patients. It demonstrates the willingness of hospital personnel to discuss their errors when provided protection from disciplinary action, as well as the feasibility of systems analysis by multidisciplinary teams.

Leape LL, Brennan TA, Laird N, Lawthers AG, et al. The nature of adverse events in hospitalized patients: Results of the Harvard Medical Practice Study II. *N Engl J Med* 1991;324:377-84.

Analysis of the types of injuries reported in the medical practice study together with analysis of causative errors.

Leape LL, Lawthers AG, Brennan TA, Johnson WG. Preventing medical injury. *QRB* 1993;8:144-149.

Description of the extent to which iatrogenic injuries reported in the medical practice study were due to errors and were, therefore, preventable.

Lesar TS, Briceland LL, Delcoure K, et al. Medication prescribing errors in a teaching hospital. *JAMA* 1990;263:2329-34.

One of the first descriptions of prescribing errors in hospitals.

Lesar TS, Briceland L, Stein DS. Factors related to errors in medication prescribing. *JAMA* 1997;277:312-317.

Results of analysis of prescribing errors detected by pharmacist review over a one-year period. Includes breakdown by type of error and related factors. Also includes related (proximal causal) factors. Ends with call for redesigning medication systems to standardize, reduce complexity and computerize them, and to integrate pharmacists with health care teams.

Massaro TA. Introducing physician order entry at a major academic medical center: I. Impact on organizational culture and behavior. *Acad Med* 1993;68:20-25.

Early description of the trials and tribulations of getting physicians to use a computerized order entry system in a teaching hospital.

McDonald CJ. Protocol-based computer reminders, the quality of care and the non-perfectibility of man. *N Eng J Med* 1976;295:1351-55.

Pioneering paper on the potential use of computerized reminders to aid medical decision-making.

McNally KM, Page MA, Sunderland VB. Failure mode and effects analysis in improving a drug distribution system. *Am J Health-Syst Pharm* 1997;54:171-177.

Description of use of FMEA in pharmacy practice.

Melmon KL. Preventable drug reactions—causes and cures. *Sem Med Beth Israel Hosp* 1971;284:1361-7.

One of the earliest papers on preventable adverse drug events. A classic.

Norman DA. *The Psychology of Everyday Things*. New York, NY: Basic Books; 1988.

A fun read, this book places everyday experiences (and frustrations) in a cognitive psychological context and includes many surprising and interesting insights. A good place to start serious reading about errors and how the mind works. Full of ideas and concepts.

Perrow C. *Normal Accidents*. New York, NY: Basic Books; 1984.

A fascinating book that opens the world of complex systems and introduces the reader to concepts of coupling and opaque systems. The contrasts between the effectiveness of error prevention in aviation and the merchant marine are striking.

Reason J. *Human Error*. New York, NY: Cambridge University Press; 1990.
The "bible" of error theory, written by the leading authority. Reason reviews the literature and establishes a theoretical framework for understanding error, based in large part on his and Rasmussen's work. A treasure of important concepts.

Wiener EL, Nagle DC, eds. *Human Factors in Aviation*. San Diego, CA: Academic Press; 1988.
Wiener is "Mr. Human Factors" for the aviation community. In this book he reviews the art and science of aviation safety.

REDUCING ADVERSE DRUG EVENTS ADDITIONAL RESOURCES

Barker KN. The effects of an experimental medication system on medication errors and costs: I. Introduction and errors study. *Am J Hosp Pharm* 1969;26:324-333.

Barker KN. The effects of an experimental medication system on medication errors and costs: II. The cost study. *Am J Hosp Pharm* 1969;26:388-397.

Barker KN, Allan EL. Research on drug-use-system errors. *Am J Health-Syst Pharm* 1995; 52:400-406.

Bates DW, Leape LL, Petrycki S. Incidence and preventability of adverse drug events in hospitalized adults. *J Gen Intern Med* 1993;8:289-94.

Brennan TA, Leape LL, Laird N, Hebert L, Localio AR, Lawthers AG, et al. Incidence of adverse events and negligence in hospitalized patients: Results of the Harvard Medical Practice Study I. *N Engl J Med* 1991; 324:370-376.

Cohen MR, Anderson RW, Attilio RM, et al. Preventing medication errors in cancer chemotherapy. *Am J Health-Syst Pharm* 1996;53:737-746.

Cook RI, Potter S, Woods DD, McDonald JS. Evaluating the human engineering of microprocessor-controlled operating room devices. *J Clin Monitoring* 1991;7:217-226.

Cook RI, Woods DD. Operating at the sharp end: The complexity of human error. In Bogner MS, ed. *Human Error in Medicine*. Hillsdale, NJ: Lawrence Erlbaum; 1994.

Cook RI, Woods DD. New technology and practitioner performance: Implication of aviation incidents involving automation for the development of total intravenous anesthesia (TIVA). *J Clin Anesth* (in press).

Cook RI, Woods DD, Howdie MB, Horrow JC, Gaba DM. Unintentional delivery of vasoactive drugs with an electromechanical infusion device. *J Cardiothor Vas Anesth* 1992;6:238-244.

Edmondson AE. Learning from mistakes is easier said than done: Group and organizational influences on the detection and correction of human error. *J Applied Behav Sci* 1996;32:5-28.

Evans RS, Pestotnik SL, Classen DC, Bass SB, Menlove RL, Gardner RM. Development of computerized adverse drug event monitor. *AMIA, Inc.* 1992;23-27.

Gaba DM. Human errors in anesthetic mishaps. *Internat Anesth Clin* 1989;27:137-147.

Gersick CJG, Hackman JR. Habitual routines in task-performing groups. *Organizational Behavior Human Decision Processes* 1990;47:65-97.

Gopher D, Olin M, Donchin Y, et al. The nature and causes of human errors in a medical intensive care unit. Proceedings of the Human Factors Society 33rd annual meeting; Oct. 18, 1989.

Hackman JR. Teams, leaders, and organizations: New directions for crew-oriented flight training. In Wiener EL, Kanki BG, Helmreich RL eds. *Cockpit Resource Management*. Orlando, FL: Academic Press; 1993.

Hackman JR, Wageman R. Total quality management: Empirical, conceptual, and practical issues. *Administrative Science Quarterly* 1995;40:309-42.

Hackman JR, Walton RE. Leading groups in organizations. In Goodman PS, ed. *Designing Effective Work Groups*. San Francisco, CA: Jossey-Bass; 1986.

Helfiker D. Facing our mistakes. *N Engl J Med* 1984;310:118-22.

Helmreich RL, Schaefer HG. Team performance in the operating room. In Bogner MS, ed. *Human Error in Medicine*. Hillside, NJ: Lawrence Erlbaum; 1994.

Massaro TA. Introducing physician order entry at a major academic medical center: II. Impact on medical education. *Acad Med* 1993; 68:25-30.

Nagel DC. Human error in aviation operations. In Wiener EL, Nagel DC, eds. *Human Factors in Aviation*. San Diego, CA: Academic Press; 1988;263-303.

Nisbett R, Ross L. *Human Inference: Strategies and Shortcomings of Social Judgment*. Englewood Cliffs, NJ: Prentice-Hall; 1980.

Rasmussen J. *Information Processing and Human-Machine Interaction*. Amsterdam: North-Holland; 1986.

Rasmussen J. Human error and the problem of causality in analysis of accidents. *Phil Trans R Soc Lond* 1990;B327:449-62.

Rasmussen J, Duncan K, Leplat J, eds. *New Technology and Human Error*. New York, NY: John Wiley and Sons; 1987.

Rasmussen J, Jensen A. Mental procedures in real-life tasks: A case study of electronic trouble-shooting. *Ergonomics* 1974;17:293-307.

Reason J. The contribution of latent human failures to the breakdown of complex systems. *Phil Trans R Soc Lond* 1990;327:475-84.

Rochlin GI, LaPorte TR, Roberts KH. The self-designing high reliability organization: Aircraft carrier flight operations at sea. *Naval War College Review* Autumn 1987;76-90.

Schaefer HG, Helmreich RL. The importance of human factors in the operating room. *Anesthes* 1994;80:479-82.

Schaefer HG, Helmreich RL, Scheidegger D. Safety in the operating theatre—Part 1: Interpersonal relationships and team performance. *Anaesth Crit Care* 1995;6:48-53.

Weinger MB, Englund CE. Ergonomic and human factors affecting anesthetic vigilance and monitoring performance in the operating room environment. *Anesthesiology* 1990;73:995-1021.

Welsh CH, Pedot R, Anderson RJ. Use of morning report to enhance adverse event detection. *J Gen Intern Med* 1996;11:454-460.

Wiener EL. Application of vigilance research: Rare, medium, or well-done? *Human Factors* 1987;29:725-736.

Wiener EL. Intervention strategies for the management of human error. *NASA CR-4547*, Ames Research Center, Moffett Field, CA; 1993.

Wiener EL, Kanki BG, Helmreich RL, eds. *Cockpit Resource Management.* San Diego, CA: Academic Press; 1993.

Woods DD, Cook RI, Billings C. The impact of technology on physician cognition and performance. *J Clin Monitor* 1995;11:5-8.

Woods DD, Johannesen L, Cook RI, Sarter N. *Behind Human Error: Cognitive Systems, Computers and Hindsight.* Dayton, OH: Crew Systems Ergonomic Information and Analysis Center; 1994.

Wu AW, Folkman S, McPhee SJ, Lo B. Do house officers learn from their mistakes? *JAMA* 1991;265:2089-2094

Institute for Safe Medication Practices (ISMP)
300 West Street Road
Warminster, PA 18974
Phone: (215) 956-9181
Fax: (215) 956-9266

The Institute for Safe Medication Practices (ISMP) is a not-for-profit organization that works closely with health care practitioners and institutions, regulatory agencies, professional organizations, and the pharmaceutical industry to provide education about adverse drug events and prevention methods. ISMP provides an independent review of medication errors that have been voluntarily submitted by practitioners to a national Medication Errors Reporting Program (MERP) operated by the U.S. Pharmacopeia (USP). All information derived from the MERP is shared with the U.S. Food and Drug Administration (FDA) and pharmaceutical companies whose products are mentioned in the reports. Information from the reports may be used by USP to impact on drug standards. The Medication Errors Reporting Program can be reached 24 hours a day at (800) 23-ERROR.

ISMP is dedicated to the sage use of medications through improvements in drug distribution, naming, packaging, labeling, and delivery system design. The organization has established a national advisory board of practitioners to assist in problem solving. ISMP is an FDA MedWatch partner and promotes the FDA's efforts to reduce adverse drug reactions.

ISMP regularly publishes information on errors and root causes of medication errors in professional journals and press reports. A biweekly fax/E-mail alert system, *ISMP Medication Safety Alert,* communicates error advisories based on recent reports submitted to the US Pharmacopeia's Medication Errors Reporting Program. USP's Practitioner Reporting Network (PRN) publishes the *USP Quality Review,* which often discusses medication error topics. The Food and Drug Administration and others also publish medication safety information. This information should be monitored and used for error prevention; the fact that an incident happened sends a strong signal that it will happen again somewhere else.

US Pharmacopeia (USP)
12601 Twinbrook Parkway
Rockville, MD 20852
Phone: (800) 4-USP-PRN [(800)-487-7776]
http://www.usp.org

USP Medication Errors Reporting Program
Phone: (800) 23-ERROR (800-233-7767)

National Coordinating Council for Medication Error Reporting and Prevention
Office of the Secretariat
USP
12601 Twinbrook Parkway
Rockville, MD 20852
Phone: (800) 822-8772

Definitions and Glossary

The need for standard terminology about error in health care is important at both the local and national level. At the work site level, common terminology fosters consistent reporting and helps to minimize confusion. If an event is regarded as an error by one person but not by another, then consistent reporting and appropriate responses are difficult. Further, management oversight of errors will be impeded if managers receive inconsistent and incomplete information.

Consistency is also needed at a macro level—any level higher than the local level, extending to national. Health care providers want to know how their error rates compare to the rates of similar facilities. Public policy makers (legislators and regulators) want to know overall error rates to set priorities for action. The local and macro needs are linked, because without consistent definitions at the local level—even assuming a good job of centrally reporting all the data—it will be impossible to create a reliable central data bank for calculating national error rates.

There is also value in describing the various types of errors in a uniform fashion. *Note:* These categories are not mutually exclusive because of the multidisciplinary nature of the medication processes.

TYPES OF MEDICATION ERRORS

Prescribing error Incorrect drug selection (based on indications, contraindications, known allergies, existing drug therapy, and other factors), dose, dosage form, quantity, route, concentration, rate of administration, or instructions for use of a drug product ordered or authorized by a physician (or other legitimate prescriber); illegible prescriptions or medication orders that lead to errors that reach the patient; use of nonstandard nomenclature or abbreviations.

Omission error The failure to administer an ordered dose to a patient before the next scheduled dose, if any. An omission error assumes there was no prescribing error. Excluded would be (1) a patient's refusal to take the medication, or (2) a decision not to administer the dose because of recognized contraindications. If an explanation for the omission is apparent (for example, the patient was away from the nursing unit for tests or medication was not available), that reason should be documented in the appropriate records.

Wrong time error Administration of medication outside a predefined time interval from its scheduled administration time (for example, 30 minutes). This interval should be established by each individual health care facility.

Unauthorized drug error Administration to the patient of medication not authorized by a legitimate prescriber for the patient. This would include, for example, a wrong drug, a dose given to the wrong patient, a dose given after the order has been discontinued, unordered drugs, and doses given outside a stated set of clinical guidelines or protocols.

Improper dose error Administration to the patient of a dose that is greater than or less than the amount ordered by the prescriber or administration to the patient of duplicate doses, that is, one or more dosage units in addition to those that were ordered.

Note: Excluded would be (1) allowable deviations based on preset ranges established by individual health care organizations in consideration of measuring devices routinely provided to those who administer drugs to patients (for example, not administering a dose based on a patient's measured temperature or blood glucose level) or other factors such as conversion of doses expressed in the apothecary system to the metric system, and (2) topical dosage forms for which medication orders are not expressed quantitatively.

TYPES OF MEDICATION ERRORS (CONTINUED)

Wrong dosage form error Administration to the patient of a drug product in a different dosage form than ordered by the prescriber.

Note: Excluded would be accepted protocols (established by the Pharmacy and Therapeutics Committee or its equivalent) that authorize pharmacists to dispense alternate dosage forms for patients with special needs (for example, liquid formulations for patients with nasogastric tubes or those who have difficulty swallowing), as allowed by state regulation.

Wrong drug preparation error Drug product incorrectly formulated or manipulated before administration. This would include, for example, incorrect dilution or reconstitution, mixing drugs that are physically or chemically incompatible, and inadequate product packaging.

Wrong administration technique error Inappropriate procedure or improper technique in the administration of a drug. This would include doses administered (1) via the wrong route (different from the route prescribed), (2) via the correct route but at the wrong site (for example, left eye instead of right), and (3) at the wrong rate of administration.

Deteriorated drug error Administration of a drug that has expired or for which the physical or chemical dosage form integrity has been compromised. This would include, for example, administration of expired drugs and improperly stored drugs.

Monitoring error Failure to review a prescribed regimen for appropriateness and detection of problems, or failure to use appropriate clinical or laboratory data for adequate assessment of patient response to prescribed therapy.

Compliance error Inappropriate patient behavior regarding adherence to a prescribed medication regimen.

SEVERITY OF ERRORS

A method for categorizing the severity of errors can be used for targeting interventions to the most serious errors. The system most commonly in use has been published in the *American Journal of Hospital Pharmacy*.

GLOSSARY

A

Adverse drug event (ADE) An injury, large or small, caused by the use (including nonuse) of a drug. It can be as harmless as a drug rash or as serious as death from an overdose. There are two types of ADEs: those caused by errors and those that occur despite proper usage. If an ADE is caused by an error it is, by definition, preventable. Nonpreventable ADEs (injury, but no error) are called adverse drug reactions (ADRs).

Adverse drug reaction (ADR) Defined by the World Health Organization to characterize injuries caused when drugs are used in the usual accepted fashion. By definition then, an ADR does not result from an error. Unfortunately, many have used this term as synonymous with ADE, which blurs an important distinction.

Adverse event An injury caused by medical treatment, not necessarily due to an error.

Affordance An attribute of equipment or work space that communicates how it is to be used without written or verbal instructions. For example, a pointed knob that is rotated to increase the signal according to an ascending scale above it.

Authority communication Communication between two or more parties where the higher authority of one person creates perceived obstacles to direct communication. The result is indirect, mitigated, or omitted communication.

B

Buffer A design characteristic that prevents errors from resulting in an accident, either by altering the process so it can proceed unimpaired, or by automatically correcting the error.

C

Constraint A limitation of the options available to keep behavior in a "safe" zone. See forcing function.

Critical pathway A series of sequential steps in a process that are required to ensure a satisfactory outcome.

D

Drive out fear A key concept in process improvement that underscores the need for all parties to be convinced that they can offer information and work on improvement without fear of punishment for acknowledging problems or errors.

E

Error An unintended act, or one that fails to achieve its intended outcome.

F

Failure mode effects analysis (FMEA) An analytic method that delineates the aspects of a system that have failed and the consequences of these. A fairly structured approach, it is used to understand the types of errors that are occurring in a system in order to remediate the system itself.

Fault tree analysis Flow chart analysis of an adverse event or error that depicts the activities that contribute to an event and their relationships to each other. Used most often to analyze the system features and confluence of events that cause errors.

Forcing function A physical constraint that prevents one from making an error. An example is not being able to start your car unless it is in the parking gear.

GLOSSARY (CONTINUED)

H

Handoff A transfer of information, materials, people, or supplies from one person to another. Examples are the various stages in processing medication orders before the pharmacist sees them (from physician to clerk to nurse to pharmacy). Slips easily happen at the transfer points.

Human factors The determinants (elements) of a task or process that result from human capacity, including memory, skill, energy, and knowledge.

L

Latent error An error of design, maintenance, training, or management that creates an unsafe situation that increases the likelihood that individuals will err. These occur proximal in time to the error actually causing an accident.

Look-alikes and sound-alikes Apparent multiple choices to accomplish one action, when only one correct behavior exists. An example is nearly identical-sounding medications, such as dobutamine and dopamine. If they are placed side by side, a staff person may take the wrong one off the shelf because the names are so similar.

M

Medication error Any error, large or small, at any point in the medication system from the time the drug is ordered until the patient receives it. This differs from some prior definitions that considered only deviations from the physician's order as errors. Since nearly half of all errors occur in the prescribing stage, these must be included in the definition. A medication error may or may not result in an adverse drug event.

Mistake An error of conscious thought; an error of intent (i.e., not thinking straight). Applied to rule-based or knowledge-based cognition.

Mitigated communication Communication that is less than direct and timely, often the result of unequal status of the parties communicating. For example, a nurse may convey information to a chief of service in an indirect way, even during a crisis or resuscitation effort, saying "Are you sure you want this dose of epinephrine?" rather than "This dose is too high."

Multiple entry Entry of the same data by more than one person in several locations, such as a physician writing an order which is then transcribed and later entered into a pharmacy computer.

N

Natural mapping When the controls or equipment or space is laid out in a way that corresponds to its natural use. An example is when the controls of a stove burner are laid out in a square that corresponds to the layout of the burners.

P

Potential adverse drug event (PADE)
A potential ADE is a serious medication error—one that has the potential to cause an ADE, but did not, either by luck (for example, the patient was not allergic to the drug despite a note in the record stating so) or because it was intercepted (for example, the nurse recognized an order for a medication to which the patient is allergic and called the physician to get it changed). Examining potential ADEs helps to identify both where the system is failing (the error) and where it is working (the interception).

Preventable adverse drug event An injury due to an error in the use of a drug (including failure to use).

Process A series of related actions to achieve a defined outcome. Ordering medication or administering medication are processes, as is administering anesthesia.

Protocols A set of rules governing a process or procedure. A protocol is usually the required procedure in a given circumstance, in contrast to a guideline, which is a recommendation.

Psychological precursors Conditions of the workplace that increase the likelihood of human error. Includes poor work schedules and double shifts, as well as poor lighting, noise, heat or cold, or other stress-producing environmental factors.

R

Redundancy Having another resource to back up a critical resource being used. For example, having a back-up heart-lung machine in the operating room or having two concurrent continuous measurements of blood pressure or oxygen.

S

Simulation A training and feedback method in which the learners actually practice the tasks or processes in lifelike circumstances using models or virtual reality, with feedback from observers, other team members, and video cameras to assist improvement of skills.

Slip An action error; an error of subconscious or automatic behavior.

System An interdependent group of processes with a common purpose.

Systems analysis Analysis of errors to identify the underlying process failures; not just the components' performance, but also how all the parts of the system fit together, communicate, and function.

T

Task A single defined activity, such as preparing a medication for administration or setting up an infusion pump. Tasks may also be broken down into component parts, but usually only involve one person.

V

Vigilance A state of being watchful and alert to danger or trouble. (The limits to human capacity for vigilance are known causes of errors.)

High-Hazard Medications: Safeguarding

A cooperative effort of the Institute for Safe Medication Practices, Warminster, PA and the Institute for Healthcare Improvement, Boston, MA

While most medications have a large margin of safety, a small number of drugs have a high risk of causing injury or fatality when they are misused. We call these "high-hazard medications" to draw attention to this characteristic so that all involved in their use will treat them with the care and respect they require. Errors may not be more common with these drugs than with any others, but the consequences of these errors can be devastating. For this reason, special attention is required. These high-hazard medications should be packaged differently, stored differently, prescribed differently, and administered differently than others. Whenever possible, "forcing functions"—methods that make it impossible for the drug to be given in a potentially lethal manner—should be developed and instituted.

Against Errors

HIGH-HAZARD MEDICATIONS TO BE TARGETED FOR SPECIFIC INTERVENTION:

1 Adrenergic agonists
2 Intravenous adrenergic antagonists
3 Amiodarone/amrinone mix-ups
4 Benzodiazepines
5 Calcium (IV)
6 Chemotherapeutic agents
7 Chloral hydrate liquid (pediatrics)
8 Heparin (IV)
9 Insulin
10 Lidocaine
11 Magnesium sulfate (IV)
12 Opiate narcotics
13 Neuromuscular blocking agents
14 Potassium chloride and potassium phosphate (IV)
15 Sodium chloride (IV), high concentrations
16 Theophylline

THREE STRATEGIES TO DECREASE THE EFFECTS OF ERRORS IN USE OF HIGH-HAZARD DRUGS

Reduce the possibility of errors

The primary means of reducing adverse drug events is prevention: Make sure that they do not occur in the first place. Prevention efforts include reducing the number of medications on formulary, reducing the number of concentrations and volumes to choose from, and removing high-hazard drugs from clinical areas.

One example is packaging oral liquids in an oral syringe whose tip is incompatible with the IV line instead of a parenteral luer lock syringe, which connects perfectly to the IV line. This makes it difficult or impossible to erroneously inject the oral liquid since the tip of the oral syringe is incompatible with the IV line.

Make errors visible

Because not all errors can be prevented, it is important to make errors visible when they do occur. One example is double checking PCA pump settings for high-hazard drugs. If an incorrect rate of infusion is programmed into a PCA pump, a second check prior to initiating the infusion will make the error visible.

Minimize the consequences of errors

It is possible to reduce the adverse effects of errors that do occur. For example, fatal errors have occurred in which the contents of 50 mL vials of lidocaine 2% were given intravenously instead of mannitol that was packaged in vials of similar appearance. If lidocaine were available only in 10 mL vials, such mistakes would not be fatal.

KEY CHANGE CONCEPTS FOR PREVENTING ERRORS IN THE USE OF HIGH-HAZARD DRUGS

The following specific suggestions incorporate the three strategies discussed above:

Use constraints and forcing functions

Clearly, the best way to prevent an error is to ensure that it is difficult or impossible to make such an error. Such a check is called a constraint (difficult) or a forcing function (impossible). An example of a constraint is permitting the use of a chemotherapeutic agent only after the order has been approved by a senior attending physician. Other useful constraints are pharmacy screening of all orders for high-hazard medications for dose limits, automatic stop orders, and dose limit protocols.

A good example of a forcing function is making a form of a drug unavailable. For example, removing vials of concentrated potassium chloride from the nursing unit makes it impossible for a nurse to accidentally rapidly infuse concentrated potassium chloride intravenously, a fatal accident that occurs 20 to 30 times annually in the United States. (To implement this change, the pharmacy must make up IV bags of diluted potassium chloride and provide them to units as needed.) Another example of a forcing function is removing a hazardous drug from the formulary if there is a safer substitute.

Use protocols and checklists

Having a detailed and explicit method for use of a medication is the best way to ensure that it will be used properly. A good protocol is easy to understand, easy to use, and comprehensive enough to ensure proper dosage. When all personnel—doctors, nurses, and pharmacists—follow protocols, a multilevel checking system is built into the process.

A good example of the value of protocols is chemotherapy, where the regimens are complicated and differ from one use to the next. A protocol can ensure that clinicians obtain adequate information (such as height and weight) and use data appropriately for calculations. (Someone still has to check and double check the calculations, however.) Protocols have also been used for heparin and coumadin.

Preprinted orders are a form of protocol that ensures standard usage. Orders can include spaces for entry of crucial data and calculations (such as chemotherapy protocols).

Avoid multiple protocols! It is important that only one protocol be available for each specific drug use. Catering to professional preferences with multiple protocols is a set-up for errors. For example, there is no need to have more than one sliding scale for insulin or more than one "K scale" (protocol for the amount of KCl—potassium chloride—to give for patients with hypokalemia).

Use distinctive labels

All hazardous drugs should bear labels that make them readily distinguishable from other medications. This communicates instantly the reminder that this drug needs special handling: "Keep your guard up!" Using a distinctive color is very effective.

At a minimum, the label on every hazardous drug should contain a warning in large print: "Caution: Overdose of this medication can cause serious injuries or death."

Another form of differentiation is to change labeling to emphasize differentiating portions of a drug name. For instance, it is much easier to differentiate DOBUTamine and DOPamine than it is to differentiate dobutamine and dopamine.

Institution-generated labels should be designed to emphasize active ingredients and minimize nonessential data. The FDA and manufacturers have set up guidelines as to size of drug name and strength.

Reduce the number of options

The more options available for any medication (multiple doses, concentrations, and volumes), the more likely it is that an error will occur. Concentrations and volumes of all available high-hazard medications should be reduced to one or two if possible. This will decrease the size of the formulary, reduce floor stocks, and reduce the possibility of errors.

For example, instead of having 2% lidocaine available in both 50 mL and 10 mL volumes, reduce the availability to one option: the 10 mL volume.

Externalize or centralize error-prone processes: Preparation of IV solutions

Preparation of IV solutions in patient care areas can be hazardous. Distractions, nonstandard concentrations, lack of nursing expertise, and erroneous calculations may all lead to errors during IV preparation of high-hazard medications such as intravenous potassium.

Most high-hazard drugs given by IV infusion are available commercially in premixed form. "Externalizing" the error-prone process of IV solution preparation from the hospital to the factory by using commercially prepared, premixed products reduces the risk of error during preparation.

Where commercial forms are not available, as in many pediatric situations, the preparation of IV solutions should be centralized to the pharmacy and not permitted on nursing units.

Use check systems

Organizations should identify error-prone processes and employ methods of error-proofing. One such method is using check systems. Examples include the following:

- The work of pharmacy technicians must be checked by pharmacists and, in critical procedures, the work of pharmacists must be checked by a second pharmacist.
- Independent checks should be made by Pain Service staff, a second nurse, or the pharmacist when setting pump rates and concentrations for patient controlled analgesia (PCA) or high-hazard drug infusions.
- In pediatrics and geriatrics and for certain high-hazard drugs, calculations should be checked independently by at least two individuals.

Use reminders

Place labels on drug containers or in drug storage locations to remind staff of potential problems. Use computer fields in drug inventory databases to flash warnings to staff during computer order entry.

Standardize dosing procedures

Calculating doses based on weight or other factors such as renal function is error-prone, particularly for vasoactive IV medications. To avoid calculation errors, use standard dosing charts or tables. These charts and tables can take multiple factors into consideration including solution concentration, patient weight, and rate of infusion. This simplifies dosing. For example, microgram/kg/minute dosing is difficult to calculate but easy to follow when based on standard dosing charts or tables. Such charts or tables can even be in the form of labels affixed to infusion containers.

What To Do Next

This Guide is full of ideas for change and examples of organizations that have tested those ideas and made real improvements in reducing adverse drug events. But knowing what changes to make and actually making them are two very different things.

The checklist that follows is designed to help you take what you have learned and put it into action.

Set an aim relative to reducing adverse drug events.

Make the aim ambitious, precise, and feasible.
Meet with senior leaders to ensure that the aim is in harmony with the organization's strategic mission and has their explicit support.

See Part 2, Setting Aims, pp. 14–17.

Form a team.

Think about the different areas that will be affected by the aim, and make sure the team has the right mix of people (system leadership, technical expertise, and day-to-day leadership) to get the job done.

See Part 2, Forming the Team, pp. 18–21.

Identify a measure and track it over time.

Measuring tells you if the changes you are testing are helping to achieve the aim. Choose a measure that relates directly to the aim and plan a simple way to collect the data.

See Part 2, Establishing Measures, pp. 22–25.

Develop a good idea for change.

Use the change concepts in Part 3 to help you come up with good ideas for changes.

See Part 3, Change Concepts for Reducing Adverse Drug Events, pp. 49–78.

Test a change on a small scale.

Remember, all improvement requires making a change. Move as quickly as possible to testing a change on a small scale.

See Part 4, Achieving Breakthrough Improvement in Reducing Adverse Drug Events, pp. 79–134, for many examples of changes tested by organizations in the Collaborative.